Glaucoma Surgical Techniques

Edited by

Richard P. Mills, MD

Department of Ophthalmology
University of Washington

Robert N. Weinreb, MD

Department of Ophthalmology
University of California, San Diego

AMERICAN ACADEMY OF OPHTHALMOLOGY

American Academy of Ophthalmology

655 Beach Street

P.O. Box 7424

San Francisco, CA 94120-7424

Library of Congress Cataloging-in-Publication Data

Glaucoma surgical techniques / edited by Richard P. Mills, Robert N.
Weinreb.
    p.   cm. — (Ophthalmology monographs ; 4)
    Includes bibliographical references.
    Includes index.
    ISBN 1-56055-008-2
    1. Glaucoma—Surgery.   I. Mills, Richard P., 1943–
II. Weinreb, Robert N., 1949–   .   III. Series.
    [DNLM: 1. Glaucoma—surgery.   W1 OP372L v. 4 / / WW 290 G55019]
RE871.G5725   1991
617.7′41—dc20
DNLM/DLC
    for Library of Congress   91-4576
                                                                CIP
Printed in MEXICO

Contributors

George Baerveldt, MD

University of Southern California

Richard A. Lewis, MD

University of California, Davis

Richard P. Mills, MD

University of Washington

Donald S. Minckler, MD

University of Southern California

J. Rigby Slight, MD

University of California, San Diego

E. Michael Van Buskirk, MD

Devers Eye Institute, Portland, Oregon

Robert N. Weinreb, MD

University of California, San Diego

Contents

Chapter 4   **BASIC TRABECULECTOMY: SURGICAL TECHNIQUE**   **22**

E. Michael Van Buskirk, MD

Chapter 5   **BASIC TRABECULECTOMY: POSTOPERATIVE CARE**   **35**

Richard A. Lewis, MD

Preface

The origin of this monograph was a Special Focus/Skills Transfer Course on glaucoma surgical techniques offered by the American Academy of Ophthalmology. For three consecutive years, 1987 to 1989, the course was given by the contributors to this volume to Academy member ophthalmologists at the Annenberg Center for Health Sciences in Palm Springs, California, and subsequently, in 1990, as a skills transfer course at the Academy's Annual Meeting in Atlanta, Georgia.

During the several iterations of the course, the faculty learned the key issues that were important to impart to the course participants, including a standard surgical technique for trabeculectomy, and the importance of discussion periods in illustrating the diversity of technique in common use. Accordingly, in this volume, each chapter is followed by from one to three commentaries from other contributors, providing tips or variations in approach or technique. The emphasis is on practical surgical technique as practiced by the authors, and the bibliographies are intended more as suggestions for further reading than as citations.

E. Michael Van Buskirk, MD, developed the core segment of the curriculum, the basic trabeculectomy, and organized the course. Dr Van Buskirk is also responsible for the development of a companion videotape, *Glaucoma Filtration Surgery: Trabeculectomy and Variations*, in the Clinical Skills Series of the Continuing Ophthalmic Video Education (COVE) program of the Academy. We are indebted to him for providing us with the opportunity to compile this monograph.

Richard P. Mills, MD
Robert N. Weinreb, MD

PART I

Basic Information

CHAPTER 1

Wound Healing in Filtration Surgery

Robert N. Weinreb, MD

Glaucoma therapy is directed at protecting the optic nerve and preserving visual function. At present, this goal is achieved by lowering intraocular pressure with either drugs or surgery.

With glaucoma filtration surgery, sclerotrabecular tissue is excised, creating a fistula through which aqueous humor drains from the anterior chamber. The aqueous humor accumulates in the subconjunctival space, forming a filtering bleb. The subconjunctival space in a functioning bleb has loosely arranged tissue with histologically clear space.

In most surgical procedures, it is desirable to enhance postoperative wound healing, a normal biologic response to tissue injury. After glaucoma filtration surgery, however, wound healing can lead to episcleral fibroproliferation and histologically dense collagenous tissue, with resulting filtration failure. To maximize the potential for a successful outcome with filtration surgery, therefore, it seems desirable to selectively inhibit the wound-healing response of scleral and episcleral tissue while simultaneously leaving conjunctival

wound healing intact. By understanding the wound-healing response, the surgeon may be able to plan a more rational approach to preoperative management, surgical techniques, and postoperative care of patients undergoing glaucoma filtration surgery.

1-1

WOUND-HEALING RESPONSE

When tissue is incised, cells (eg, conjunctival epithelium or scleral fibroblasts), extracellular matrix, and blood vessels are damaged and disrupted. Repair starts almost immediately after injury, when a number of growth factors in serum, secondary aqueous humor, and cellular extracts are released into the injured area. The wound-healing response consists of a sequence of programmed steps, each of which contributes to the restoration of structural and functional integrity of the tissue.

Wound healing can be considered to occur in three overlapping phases (Figure 1-1). First, cellular migration and inflammation occur immediately after injury and predominate for several days. Growth factors are thought to play important roles during this phase not only as mitogens but as chemoattractants, which recruit leukocytes and fibroblasts to the injured area. Next, cells proliferate, particularly fibroblasts, with biosynthesis of new extracellular material and wound contraction. This phase may predominate for several weeks and leads to formation of granulation tissue. Proliferation of cells within the wound may be determined by the kinds and levels of growth factors present. During the third phase of wound healing, this tissue is remodeled over several months— a process that involves collagen biosynthesis, crosslinking, and degradation.

1-1-1 Inflammation Phase

Within 1 day, a clot consisting of platelets, fibrin, fibronectin, and polymorphonuclear leukocytes (PMNs) is apparent within a sutured wound of vascularized tissue (eg, conjunctiva or episclera). The clot can be considered to be the result of biochemical activation, which involves the translation of mechanical injury into biochemical signals. Tissue injury, blood, and possibly aqueous humor are each associated with the accumulation of growth factors in the wound. These growth factors may contribute to initiating the cascade of the wound-healing response. For several days, the number of PMNs increases. In conjunctiva, this increase is accompanied by epithelial cell migration, which covers the wound surface. After a few days, the tissue increases in thickness and the number of mononuclear cells increases, with fewer

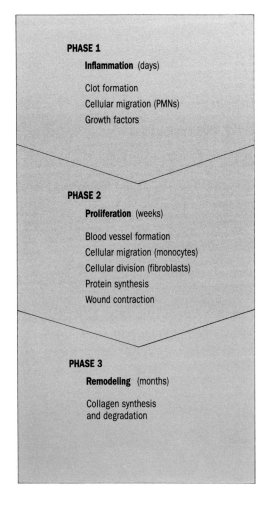

Figure 1-1 *Major events in wound healing. Wound healing can be considered to be a cascade of events with three overlapping phases. After injury, cellular migration and inflammation occur. Next, cells proliferate with biosynthesis of new extracellular material and wound contraction. Finally, the tissue is remodeled during the third phase.*

PMNs. Because inflammation appears to be an essential event for normal wound healing, the inhibition of wound healing may be possible with the use of anti-inflammatory agents. Without inflammation, there is no wound healing.

1-1-2 Proliferation Phase

Within a few days after injury, the number of new fibroblasts, monocytes, and blood vessels in a wound increases. During this period of biochemical amplification and cellular response, they migrate into the fibrin meshwork of the clot. The appearance of this newly formed tissue is similar to that seen in granulation tissue. In a cynomolgus monkey model of glaucoma filtration surgery, cellular proliferation is already occurring between 24 and 48 hours after surgery, peaks between 3 and 5 days, and returns to baseline by 11 days. With poorly apposed conjunctival or subconjunctival tissue, this phase may be exaggerated, with an unsightly and irritating scar. Many of the fibroblasts have considerable actin and myosin microfilaments (myofibroblasts), which enable them to contract and bring the edges of the wound together. The bridging of wound edges by the proliferation of fibroblasts, small blood vessels, and chronic inflammatory cells is accompanied by wound closure within several days of injury.

Low oxygen tension, decreased pH, and elevated lactate levels can also be found during the first several weeks, possibly as the result of increased cellular metabolism and a relative decrease in blood supply. Collagen deposition increases and the fibrin clot begins to resolve during this phase. Monocytes, which assist PMNs in host defense, are probably the major source of locally acting growth factors at this time and direct repair until the wound is healed. Also, it has been speculated that there are quantitative or qualitative differences in growth factors in aqueous humor that may have clinical significance. Pharmacologic agents or other therapeutic adjuncts that can inhibit fibroproliferation or wound contraction during this phase can directly affect the wound-healing response.

1-1-3 Remodeling Phase

Proteolytic enzymes can be found in a wound early during the postoperative period. They are derived in part from the circulation and from PMNs and monocytes; aqueous humor may also be a source. These enzymes aid in digesting cellular debris and the clot. At the same time, the newly formed fibroblasts actively biosynthesize collagen, glycosaminoglycans, and elastins. In normal wound healing, newly biosynthesized collagen is initially deposited irregularly within the wound. Glycosaminoglycans may facilitate the spatial arrangement of proliferating cells and newly deposited collagen fibrils and may contribute to metabolic regulation in the wound. As collagen biosynthesis increases, wound mass also increases.

As early as 2 weeks after injury, the wound begins to undergo a remodeling process in which the young, irregularly deposited collagen is gradually replaced over a period of months by collagen that imparts tensile strength approximately equal to that of normal tissue. This remodeling is characterized initially by large quantities of collagenase, biosynthesized primarily by mononuclear leukocytes. Thus, an equilibrium is established in which collagen biosynthesis and degradation are balanced; although the collagen is changing in quality, it is not increasing in quantity. During vitamin C deficiency, collagen biosynthesis is altered, impairing wound healing. Agents that inhibit collagen crosslinking, such as beta-aminoproprionitrile, can be employed to pharmacologically inhibit this stage of the wound-healing process.

1-2

GENERAL PRINCIPLES

If the conceptualization of wound healing described above is correct, certain principles should lead to a more rational approach to preoperative management, surgical techniques, and postoperative care of patients undergoing glaucoma filtration surgery:

1. Without inflammation, wound healing does not take place. Hence, preoperative and postoperative inflammation should be minimized by treatment with an anti-inflammatory agent, such as a corticosteroid. Topical, and even systemic, corticosteroids can be administered frequently. The effectiveness of topical and systemic nonsteroidal agents is not known.

2. Disruption of the blood–aqueous barrier causes protein (including growth factors) and cells to leak into the anterior chamber. Hence, potent cholinesterase inhibitors, such as echothiophate iodide, should be discontinued 2 weeks before surgery. These agents have a tendency to disrupt the blood–aqueous barrier and may facilitate postoperative inflammation.

3. Besides deepening the anterior chamber of a phakic eye, cycloplegic agents, such as atropine, may enhance the integrity of the blood–aqueous barrier. Their administration may reduce postoperative inflammation and leakage of plasma proteins into the eye.

4. Tissue trauma, which increases inflammation, should be minimized, and unnecessary manipulation of tissue avoided. In this regard, meticulous dissection of conjunctival tissue should be undertaken to avoid buttonhole formation.

5. Numerous growth factors, which can initiate inflammation, are brought into the surgical wound when blood is present. Hence, hemostasis should be obtained throughout the surgical procedure.

6. Clean surgical incisions heal optimally and with minimal granulation tissue when closed properly. Therefore, wound edges of incised conjunctiva, Tenon's capsule, and sclera should be carefully reapproximated with a low-reactive suture material and a fine needle to avoid excessive fibro-proliferation.

7. Pharmacologic intervention with agents capable of influencing the various phases of the wound-healing response may promote filtration success. Timing the administration of these agents is probably critical. For example, early during the inflammatory response, it may be most appropriate to use corticosteriods intensively to reduce inflammation. Antiproliferative agents, such as 5-fluorouracil (to inhibit fibroproliferation) and colchicine (to inhibit wound contraction), may be most effective during the second phase of wound healing. Restricting the use of antiproliferative agents in humans to a brief, discrete period of cellular proliferation may be optimal. Angiogenesis inhibitors may also be particularly effective during this stage to inhibit the growth of new blood vessels. Drugs that interfere with the remodeling phase, such as the collagen crosslinking inhibitor beta-aminoproprionitrile, may have greatest benefit during the several months following surgery.

1-3

SUMMARY

Further characterization of the wound-healing response and its chemotherapeutic modification after glaucoma filtration surgery may lead to improved surgical success.

BIBLIOGRAPHY

Barbul A, Pines E, Caldwell M, et al, eds: *Growth Factors and Other Aspects of Wound Healing.* New York: Alan R. Liss; 1988.

Howes EL: Basic mechanisms in pathology. In Spencer W, ed: *Ophthalmic Pathology: An Atlas and Textbook.* Philadelphia: WB Saunders Co; 1985;1:43–51.

Skuta GL, Parrish RK II: Wound healing in glaucoma filtering surgery. *Surv Ophthalmol* 1987;**32**:149–170.

Weinreb RN, Mantzioros N: Modulation of surgical wound healing in glaucoma filtering surgery. In Drance SM, Van Buskirk EM, Neufeld AH, eds: *Applied Pharmacology of Glaucoma.* Baltimore, MD: Williams & Wilkins. In press.

Commentary

Richard P. Mills, MD

The division of the normal wound-healing response into three overlapping phases—inflammation, proliferation, and remodeling—is a useful device for understanding a complicated process. Knowledge of the interplay of humoral and cellular factors in wound healing is expanding rapidly, but is still fragmentary. From a clinical perspective, a few additional points deserve emphasis:

1. The names of the three phases, chosen to describe the dominant tissue response, should not obscure the fact that many different events are occurring simultaneously during each phase. For example, during the proliferative phase, in addition to cell division, protein synthesis and collagen deposition are proceeding at a rapid rate.

2. The first, or inflammatory, phase is an acute process characterized by clot formation and cellular migration. It should not be confused with the clinical appearance of inflammation, with hyperemia and edema, which may be evident until well into the remodeling phase.

3. Standard glaucoma filtration surgery poses some ambivalence about wound healing. On the one hand, inhibition of healing of the scleral fistula is wanted so that filtration may continue; on the other hand, the overlying conjunctiva must heal to form a bleb and avoid a wound leak through which bacteria can travel unimpeded. The odds of achieving these cross-purposes can be improved if conjunctival closure is meticulous and fluid-tight while the scleral closure is loose enough to allow free aqueous flow. If drugs are used to modify wound healing, they must be titrated to suit the individual patient's conjunctival vs scleral healing response. Most desirable of all would be a surgical technique that requires no conjunctival incision; several are under development but have not yet passed the test of time.

4. Surgical techniques that minimize tissue trauma, hemorrhage, and breakdown of the blood–aqueous barrier will also reduce inflammation and enhance the success of filtration. Future surgical developments, especially with new laser technology, may prove less traumatic than current techniques.

CHAPTER 2

Surgical Anatomy of the Limbus

Donald S. Minckler, MD

This chapter discusses those anatomic features of the anterior segment of the human eye important to glaucoma filtration surgery. Most glaucoma filtration procedures, including both full-thickness procedures and trabeculectomies, are placed in the superior quadrants, beneath the upper lid. This location has multiple advantages: ease of surgical approach, more space for elevated blebs, better lubrication and protection, less long-term risk of infection, and less likelihood of diplopia from the iridectomy. Though less desirable, it is sometimes necessary to perform filtration surgery in one of the inferior quadrants, to avoid scarred conjunctiva from previous surgical procedures. Because a subsequent filtration procedure may be necessary, it is desirable to center the initial surgery in one or the other upper quadrant and spare the opposite upper quadrant for later use. The upper nasal quadrant should be given preference for the first filtration procedure in phakic eyes to facilitate the temporal rotation of a subsequent cataract incision and the avoidance of the filtration bleb (Figure 2-1).

The preoperative evaluation of patients for whom filtration surgery is contemplated should include inspection of the conjunctiva, eyelids, and lacrimal drainage apparatus to ensure that diseases of those structures, especially acute or chronic infection, will not endanger the postoperative course or preclude a favorable result.

2-1

GROSS ANATOMY

Major anatomic landmarks of the eye important to this discussion include the junction between conjunctival and corneal epithelium, the insertion of the rectus muscles, the fusion of Tenon's capsule with episclera, and the blue limbus. The normal presence of micropannus, especially at the superior corneal margin in normal adult eyes, renders the clear cornea slightly elliptical horizontally and accounts for normal variation in the width of the surgical limbus around its circumference. Normal eyes of infants and young children have no or less obvious micropannus and more round-appearing corneas.

The junction between corneal and conjunctival epithelium corresponds to the transition from mobile conjunctiva to immobile corneal epithelium. The tethering of the surface epithelium at the end of Bowman's membrane limits the elevation

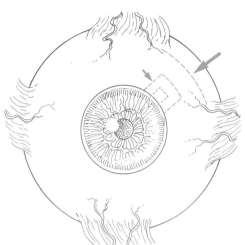

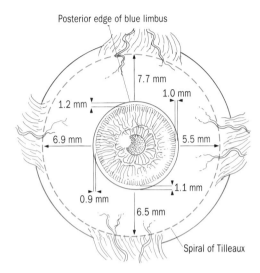

of a limbus-based conjunctival flap. An abrupt change in the radius of curvature occurs at the junction between cornea and conjunctiva, creating the external scleral sulcus, often noted during dissection of a limbus-based conjunctival flap as a slight depression at the outer edge of Bowman's membrane.

Tenon's capsule, which is usually a distinct layer easily separable from overlying conjunctiva 6 to 8 mm posterior to the limbus, fuses with the episclera about 2 mm posterior to the margin of the cornea. The variable sparsity of Tenon's capsule between its episcleral insertion and the edge of the cornea in adults may account for the development of some thin-walled blebs in a narrow zone along the corneal margin. Infants' and children's eyes generally have a prominent Tenon's capsule.

Large anterior ciliary vessels mark the insertions of the rectus muscles, including two arteries in each insertion except for the lateral rectus, which has only one (Figure 2-2).

Figure 2-1 *(Left) Anterior view of the right eye showing the preferred location of a limbus-based conjunctival Tenon's capsule incision (large arrow) and a scleral flap for trabeculectomy (small arrow). The approximate size and location of the deep scleral excision and the iridectomy are also indicated.*
Modified by permission from Minckler DS: Anatomy in glaucoma-related surgery. In: Waltman SR, et al, eds: Surgery of the Eye. *New York: Churchill Livingstone; 1988;1:311–322.*

Figure 2-2 *(Right) Anterior view of the right eye. The spiral of Tilleaux, connecting the rectus muscle insertions externally, corresponds to the ora serrata internally and marks the posterior end of the pars plana. The surgical limbus—the space between the cornea and the posterior edge of the blue limbus—is widest superiorly.*
Modified by permission from Minckler DS: Anatomy in glaucoma-related surgery. In: Waltman SR, et al, eds: Surgery of the Eye. *New York: Churchill Livingstone; 1988;1:311–322.*

Figure 2-3 *The surgical limbus and major landmarks relevant to glaucoma surgery.* Modified by permission from Minckler DS: Anatomy in glaucoma-related surgery. In: Waltman SR, et al, eds: Surgery of the Eye. *New York: Churchill Livingstone; 1988;1:311–322.*

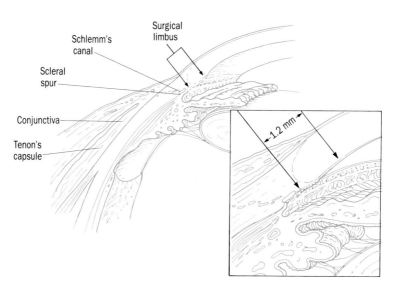

The blue limbus, widest superiorly, is a dependable landmark and clearly visible in most adult eyes. A full-thickness incision perpendicular to the posterior edge of the limbus will intersect the anterior trabecular meshwork in 75% of normal adult eyes (Figure 2-3). Because the blue limbus is less obvious in normal infants' or children's eyes, the surgeon must depend on other landmarks for orientation, such as the edge of Bowman's membrane (where the corneal and conjunctival epithelium fuse).

2-2

SURGICAL ANATOMY

The surgical limbus is bounded by a line between the ends of Bowman's and Descemet's membranes and a line perpendicular to the conjunctival epithelium extending into the iris recess. The posterior edge of the surgical limbus corresponds in all quadrants to the posterior edge of the blue limbus. The surgical limbus as defined here averages about 1.2 mm in width in the superior quadrants. Inferiorly, it is a little narrower, and directly nasally and temporally, it measures only 0.9 mm. The posterior margin of the blue limbus will recede posteriorly during dissection of a limbus-based scleral flap, corresponding to thinning of the sclera over the internal scleral sulcus in which the trabecular meshwork and Schlemm's canal reside.

During trabeculectomy with dissection of a partial-thickness limbus-based scleral flap beginning 4 to 5 mm posterior to the limbus, the bed of the dissection will initially be homogeneous and gray–white in color. Beginning about 1.5 to 2.0 mm from the limbus, the lamellar architecture of the sclera becomes more loose and aqueous veins may be encountered. As the internal scleral sulcus is unroofed and Schlemm's canal partly uncovered, the color of the bed will darken slightly. A distinctly darker demarcation line paralleling the limbus usually marks the scleral spur. A transition to clear cornea occurs at Schwalbe's line. The most certain orientation anatomically during trabeculectomy is obtained by external rotation of the deep scleral flap before excision along its posterior margin and direct viewing of the meshwork and spur on its inner surface.

Variations in infants' and children's eyes include less obvious transitions in color as the dissection crosses over Schlemm's canal and the scleral spur. The texture of the perilimbal sclera in young eyes is looser and more delicate than in adults. Inadvertent penetration of the sclera (dissection into the ciliary body) or premature perforation into the anterior chamber is more likely in young eyes than in adult eyes because the tissues are thinner and more fragile. Maturation and growth of the anterior chamber angle and the anatomic relationships between the various structures (iris, angle recess, scleral spur) are not normally completed until 6 to 12 months of age. Anatomic relationships in eyes with congenital glaucoma associated with anomalous formation of angle structures or buphthalmos may be grossly distorted and customary landmarks useless. Trabeculotomy, for example, in young eyes with corneal diameters of 14 mm or more is often complicated by the inability to clearly identify Schlemm's canal.

2-2-1 Vessels

Besides the large arteries and veins in the rectus muscle insertions, variable arrays of episcleral vessels are present in the perilimbal area. These may be massive in eyes that have been treated with vasoactive agents over a substantial period of time or that have been subjected to previous surgery. Most of the bleeding encountered during preparation of conjunctival flaps comes from episcleral vessels ruptured during dissection. Cautery of episcleral vessels should be minimal to avoid scleral shrinkage. Cautery of the scleral flap should be avoided if possible to prevent shrinkage. Cautery of the conjunctival edges should also be avoided because of potential wound leak.

Nerve loops of Axenfeld, most common nasally, mark the junction of pars plicata and pars plana internally and include vessels that may bleed profusely when cut. Preoperative use of epinephrine agents, strong miotics, aspirin, and anticoagulants can increase bleeding during filtration surgery. Ideally, epinephrine agents (including dipivefrin) should be discontinued 3 to 4 weeks prior to surgery, and systemic agents that affect bleeding and clotting time discontinued or modified with medical consultation.

2-2-2 Iris and Choroid

Normal iris vessels usually do not bleed after iridectomy. Bleeding from rubeotic iris vessels may be massive, often when intraocular pressure is suddenly lowered by paracentesis even without direct manipulation. Bleeding from the anterior edge of the ciliary body or the posterior aspect of the deep scleral excision may be substantial but will often stop with simple compression. Cautery should be used with caution to avoid inadvertent lens or zonular injury.

The choroid includes the choriocapillaris immediately external to Bruch's membrane and several layers of increasingly large venous channels. The arterial supply of blood flows into the choriocapillaris from branches of the short posterior ciliary arteries through perpendicularly oriented arterioles that are central in the lobules of the choriocapillaris. Shearing of these arterioles during surgical manipulation or distortion of the eye wall may explain intraoperative arterial choroidal hemorrhage. Venous hemorrhage in the choroid is probably the result of venous congestion triggered by hypotony during surgery and scissoring of the vortex veins by the sclera. Choroidal hemorrhage expands primarily in the suprachoroidal space adjacent to the inner scleral wall but may rupture through Bruch's membrane into the subpigment epithelial space and vitreous cavity.

Incisions into the suprachoroidal space to drain effusions can be safely made in phakic eyes 4 mm posterior to the limbus, usually centered in the inferior quadrants. In aphakic or pseudophakic eyes, a site 3 mm posterior to the limbus is preferable. Drainage sites should avoid the long posterior ciliary arteries, which invariably run forward to the ciliary body in the horizontal meridians at the 3- and 9-o'clock positions.

2-3

SUMMARY

The glaucoma surgeon must have a clear understanding of many details of anterior segment anatomy, especially the limbal landmarks that guide the placement of incisions. Localization of the scleral spur, the canal of Schlemm, and the trabecular meshwork during the dissection must be reasonably precise to ensure proper placement of the drainage fistula and to avoid complications.

BIBLIOGRAPHY

Minckler DS: Anatomy in glaucoma-related surgery. In: Herschler J, ed: *Surgery of the Eye.* New York: Churchill Livingstone; 1988;**1:** 311–322.

Hoskins HD, Kass M: *Becker-Shaffer's Diagnosis and Therapy of the Glaucomas.* 6th ed. St Louis: CV Mosby Co; 1989:372.

Van Buskirk EM: The anatomy of the limbus. *Eye* 1989;**3:**101–108.

Commentary

Richard P. Mills, MD

An understanding of the anatomic features of the surgical limbus is critical to the performance of successful filtration surgery. If possible, the surgeon should arrange with a local eye bank to obtain a donor eye that is unsuitable for corneal transplantation and spend a few minutes examining it under the operating microscope. The surgeon should fashion a superficial scleral flap, then make a full-thickness radial incision across the limbus through the dissected area and examine it end-on. Many of the anatomic features described in this chapter will take on new meaning and will be directly applicable to actual surgical situations:

1. The width of the surgical limbus, while histologically only 25% narrower at the 3- and 9-o'clock positions than at the 12-o'clock position, seems much more crowded during surgical dissection in the horizontal meridians. The conjunctival insertion is more posterior, Tenon's capsule inserts more anteriorly, and the blue zone is foreshortened. The natural tendency is to operate in an easier area, so filtration surgeries, intended to be centered in the superonasal quadrant, tend to creep toward the 12-o'clock position. If a good bleb results and cataract extraction is needed later, it is difficult to place the incision temporal enough to avoid the bleb. The surgeon's comfort level while operating away from the 12-o'clock position is increased by the knowledge that incisions perpendicular to the sclera at the posterior edge of the blue zone, even where the limbus is narrow in the horizontal meridians, will enter at, or anterior to, the trabecular meshwork.

2. Half-thickness scleral flap dissections encounter the blue zone more posteriorly than expected on the basis of inspecting full-thickness sclera at the limbus. As Figure 2-3 shows, a wedge of clearer corneal tissue extends into sclera most posteriorly at the midpoint of scleral thickness. It is important to continue the surgical dissection well forward into totally clear cornea so that the deep tissues can be excised anteriorly enough.

3. Because of the abrupt change in the radius of curvature at the limbus, lamellar dissections that do not change their angulation upon encountering this curvature change will dive deep and tend to enter the anterior chamber prematurely.

Commentary

E. Michael Van Buskirk, MD

A thorough understanding of surgical anatomy underlies successful filtration surgery. Many of the most common errors during trabeculectomy surgery derive from misinterpretation of anatomic landmarks. As Dr Minckler points out, the surgeon should bear in mind that the blue-zone transition from white sclera to clear cornea is displaced posteriorly when viewed under the partial-thickness scleral flap than when viewed directly under the conjunctiva. This occurs because the sclera–cornea interface is oblique, with the scleral portion relatively more anterior and closer to the external surface than the internal surface of the globe. This is particularly true in the vertical meridians. The obliqueness of the transition zone is much less as the operative site is shifted toward the horizontal meridians. It is also greater superiorly than inferiorly. Hence, the surgeon who elects to place a filtration fistula inferiorly should remember that the surgical blue zone will be narrower, with less margin for error.

When dissecting a half-thickness scleral flap, I find that the homogeneous gray–white color of the scleral portion of the bed gives way to a relatively well-defined, more densely white line that roughly corresponds to scleral spur. The transition to clear cornea overlying Schwalbe's line is somewhat more variable. If the surgeon advances the flap until clear cornea is encountered and then makes the fistula just posterior to the edge of clear cornea, it will be properly placed. Placing the fistula too posteriorly is one of the most common errors resulting from inadequate consideration of limbal anatomy.

CHAPTER 3

Indications, Contraindications, and Preoperative Evaluation

Richard P. Mills, MD

All types of filtration surgery involve the formation of a fistula to drain aqueous humor from the interior of the eye to the outside. As a result, the eye becomes decompressed, usually suddenly and often protractedly. Hemorrhage, macular edema, cataract, and infection may complicate the procedure and significantly compromise the patient's vision, so the decision to proceed should not be taken lightly.

Despite these potential complications, some surgeons have fueled controversy by contending that filtration surgery should be done as the initial therapeutic measure in the treatment of primary open-angle glaucoma. They cite compliance problems with medical regimens, side effects and cost of medication, and visual deterioration in spite of medication as reasons to reject medical therapy as initial treatment.

3-1

INDICATIONS

The prevailing view among American ophthalmologists is that the potential complications of filtration surgery are serious enough that other therapeutic modalities should be employed first, and incisional surgery performed only when medical therapy and laser surgery have failed (*Primary Open-Angle Glaucoma* 1989). In other words, an adequate surgical indication must be present. For most ophthalmic surgeons, the indication is as follows: *A patient with glaucoma on maximum tolerable medical therapy who has had maximal laser benefit and whose optic nerve function is failing or is likely to fail.*

3-1-1 A Patient With Glaucoma

First, the surgeon must be certain the patient has glaucoma, and not just ocular hypertension or something else. This determination implies characteristic damage to the optic nerve, visual field, or both.

Among the indicators of progressive optic nerve damage is a splinter hemorrhage at the disc margin. The surgeon must specifically look for it during each followup disc examination. Cursory inspection might easily mistake a disc hemorrhage as a retinal blood vessel because it often begins near a major retinal vessel and is oriented radially across the disc margin. However, disc hemorrhages terminate abruptly, whereas retinal vessels do not. Of course, disc hemorrhages are not unique to glaucoma, but may be found in other optic neuropathies.

Another indicator of progressive optic nerve damage is a change in either the optic cup or the neuroretinal rim. A notch in the neuroretinal rim is a reliable indicator of significant disc damage. Frequently, interval changes in the disc are very subtle and can be appreciated only by careful stereoscopic inspection with the slit lamp and funduscopic contact lens, +60- or +90-diopter handheld lens, or Hruby lens. Stereophotographs or careful drawings done at the baseline visit can be invaluable to the clinician trying to evaluate change at a subsequent examination. Monocular direct ophthalmoscopy is seldom sensitive enough to detect small interval changes. A documented change in the optic cup is an indicator that the patient has glaucoma, even if the cup size is not frankly glaucomatous.

Finally, examination of the peripapillary nerve fiber layer with red-free light is an indispensable adjunct to optic disc evaluation. A wedge-shaped defect is an indication of focal axonal damage. In glaucoma, the nerve fiber layer can also be seen to be diffusely thinned, with enhanced visibility of the retinal blood vessels caused by the loss of the overlying screen of nerve fibers. Vessel walls, particularly small- to medium-caliber ones, running perpendicular to the direction of the nerve fibers, look as though they were drawn on the surface of the retina by a pen, as opposed to being broken up into a dotted line by crossing nerve fibers. This appearance is enhanced in the larger vessels by the additional light reflex paralleling the vessel wall provided by the internal limiting membrane as it drapes over the vessel that lies on top of, rather than being embedded in, the inner retinal layers.

Comparing vessel visibility in the superior and inferior fundus in one eye or corresponding locations in both eyes is a sensitive way to detect thinning of the nerve fiber layer. Focal or generalized defects of the nerve fiber layer are corroborative evidence of disc damage, even when the disc damage is not identified.

Focal glaucomatous visual field defects, when they are arcuate or nasal step defects, are discerned readily with Goldmann manual or automated threshold perimetry. But they are not the most common kind of glaucoma field defect. In fact, generalized visual field loss is probably the most common of the glaucomatous field defects. The problem is that generalized loss of sensitivity is not pathognomonic for glaucoma. Patient factors such as fatigue, reliability, and learning effect can produce an identical generalized depression. Cataract, corneal or other media opacities, and miotic pupils can be responsible, too. Still, if these factors can be excluded, then glaucoma is to be seriously considered.

3-1-2 On Maximum Tolerable Medical Therapy

Unless contraindicated, not tolerated, or proven ineffective in the patient, a beta blocker (timolol, levobunolol, or betaxolol) should be among the medications. Betaxolol may be a little less effective than timolol or levobunolol in lowering intraocular pressure in some patients, but it has fewer side effects. Maximum medication should also include 4% pilocarpine (6% in blacks, according to Harris and Galin 1971) or its equivalent, 3% carbachol; an aphakic eye should be treated with a cholinesterase inhibitor such as 0.25% echothiophate iodide. The third type of topically administered drug is 1% dipivefrin or 2% epinephrine. Finally, an oral carbonic anhydrase inhibitor should be used or at least offered prior to a filtration surgery decision.

The word *tolerable* is open to considerable interpretation. Some of the reasons a medication would be considered intolerable are based on the ophthalmologist's judgment. Obviously, a drug should not be used if contraindicated, such as when the patient has a history of bronchial asthma and should not be given a nonselective beta blocker. If on a prior trial a given medication failed to show a measurable effect on intraocular pressure, there would be no reason to try it again. Medications such as dipivefrin and pilocarpine,

which can be used in one eye without affecting the fellow eye, can be tried so that the intraocular pressure difference between the eyes attributable to the drug can be measured.

A medication may be intolerable because of severe side effects, for example, blurred vision from pilocarpine, paresthesias from acetazolamide, and systemic effects of beta blockers. And of course, a patient's inability to comply with the drug regimen cannot be counteracted very well. Obviously, a patient whose intraocular pressure is well controlled when the patient is under continual surveillance, but who is noncompliant most of the time at home—who can't remember to use eyedrops, even after urging by physician and family—ought to be considered for laser or filtration surgery.

One point to remember in considering maximum tolerable medication is that many more medication choices exist at present than in the past. If the physician waits before changing medication until the patient loses some more visual field, then the patient may lose vision entirely before the ophthalmologist has tried all possible medications. So it is important to set up an intraocular pressure goal for the patient. If previously progressive optic nerve damage has occurred at a mean pressure of 20 mm Hg, it might be advisable to aim for a mean pressure of 16 mm Hg, continuing to add medication until that level is reached rather than waiting at each step along the way for visual deterioration.

Some reasons patients give for not using a medication really do not qualify as intolerable. For instance, a patient simply may not like to use eyedrops because they sting and burn, but will use them if informed of the importance of doing so. Some patients do not like the idea of long-term medication, and others seem to prefer any "new" or "high tech" solution. Pilocarpine blur in a young patient might make the medication intolerable as drops, but a trial of Ocuserts or pilocarpine gel might be successful. Many young patients do quite well with these alternative forms of drug delivery, and the myopia induced is stable enough that a new pair of glasses will correct it throughout the day. Nausea with acetazolamide can often be avoided by using methazolamide, which has a lower incidence of gastrointestinal side effects. Financial reasons often represent a major factor in the patient not complying with the medication regimen. For medically indigent patients who don't qualify for Medicaid, some programs sponsored by various drug companies can provide medication at reduced cost.

Detecting the noncompliant patient is a very difficult task, and one that ophthalmologists do rather poorly. In many instances, patients in the first few visits admit they haven't been using their medication as directed. So the ophthalmologist and support staff carefully instruct, encourage, and educate these patients each time, even attempting to use fear as a motivator. On later visits, noncompliant patients may say they are using a medication as prescribed because they don't want to be harassed about it anymore.

3-1-3 Who Has Had Maximal Laser Benefit

This phrase is intended to connote that 360° of anterior chamber angle has been treated by an ophthalmologist using proper treatment parameters. It is helpful to review medical records to confirm that the parameters were appropriate and that the full circumference was treated. If a patient received laser surgery when it was a new technique and when gonioscopic skills were not as widely practiced as they are today, laser applications may not have been made on the anterior trabecular meshwork as is currently recommended. Apart from that exception, re-treatment is seldom required. On the other hand, re-treatment can always be tried, at the cost of additional time and with a reduced level of expectation for success, before proceeding to filtration surgery.

Ironically, "maximal laser benefit" has been achieved in some patients on whom the laser has not been used at all. Certain kinds of glaucoma tend to respond poorly to laser surgery: developmental glaucoma, glaucoma secondary to uveitis, 360° angle recession, and chronically closed angles. Laser surgery may be used in patients with these glaucoma types, especially if the clinician believes a component of open-angle glaucoma is contributing to the disease, but the incidence of unchanged or increased intraocular pressure following the procedure is higher than with other types of glaucoma. Most of these types of glaucoma with a poor prognosis occur in the younger patient population. On the other hand, the elderly patient who has a component of trabecular meshwork aging will often respond favorably to laser surgery.

If the patient cannot cooperate or hold a steady position at the laser or if the cornea is cloudy and the laser energy is absorbed before it reaches the angle, then laser surgery is not a prerequisite of filtration surgery. If the patient has had a minimal intraocular pressure response from treatment of the first 180° of angle, it may be worthwhile to finish the second half before deciding that the laser has been of no value. But if one eye simply does not respond at all with a full 360° of treatment and the two eyes are anatomically similar, then it is probably not useful to try it in the second eye.

3-1-4 And Whose Optic Nerve Function Is Failing or Is Likely to Fail

Obviously, loss of some optic nerve function is central to the diagnosis of glaucoma in the first place. If further deterioration in visual field or if optic nerve cupping can be documented in spite of medical and/or laser treatment, then filtration surgery is indicated. But equally important is the *likelihood* of a failing optic nerve. For example, a patient's visual field is likely to deteriorate if the tension is too high for the stage of the disease (remembering that the more advanced the glaucoma, the more compulsive one needs to be about pressure control). The intraocular pressure level needed for control (the "target" pressure) is often lower in patients with advanced disease than in those with early damage (Grant and Burke 1982).

If the patient or family members have rapidly progressive damage or damage at a low intraocular pressure, an aggressive surgical approach may be justified. Consequently, patients who have gone blind from glaucoma in one eye in spite of good medical management and those with a strong family history of blindness from glaucoma are candidates for filtration surgery earlier than would otherwise be the case.

3-2

CONTRAINDICATIONS

Some contraindications to filtration surgery exist. A blind painful eye is an obvious one. No visual result is to be gained, and pain control is more expeditiously achieved through other means. Filtration surgery is also contraindicated for a blind painless eye. Because vision cannot be improved, the only result possible is to convert the eye into the blind painful category. Other contraindications to filtration surgery include ocular neoplasms, because of the risk of facilitating metastatic spread, and poor personal hygiene, with an increased risk of endophthalmitis over time. In such cases, cyclodestructive procedures should be considered as an alternative to filtration surgery.

Patients with active rubeosis iridis and neovascular glaucoma usually bleed during surgery and during the postoperative period. The resultant hyphema in the anterior chamber may take quite a while to clear. Preoperative panretinal photocoagulation and/or peripheral retinal cryotherapy is preferable to induce the neovascularization to regress, and perhaps reduce the tendency to subsequent fibrovascular proliferation. After 10 to 14 days, filtration surgery has a much improved chance of success.

3-3

PREOPERATIVE EVALUATION

During a preoperative workup, it is important to be alert to factors that increase the risks associated with filtration surgery. Systemic conditions that prevent proper patient positioning for surgery or that may be adversely affected by the stresses of surgery even under local anesthesia (eg, very recent myocardial infarction) must be detected. Other medical conditions worthy of note include diabetes, hypertension, and long-term use of systemic steroids.

Ocular conditions such as nanophthalmos or choroidal hemangioma may predispose to choroidal effusion and/or hemorrhage either intraoperatively or postoperatively, with potentially disastrous results. Averting intraoperative and postoperative complications is the responsibility of the surgeon, and adequate preoperative evaluation is necessary to avoid them.

3-4

SUMMARY

The indications for surgery discussed in this chapter are not absolute. They represent only the current prevailing view among American ophthalmologists who care for the "average" glaucoma patient. Individual patient variations frequently alter these indications (*Quality of Ophthalmic Care* 1988). Moreover, ophthalmic practice is continuously evolving, so that indications change with time as new knowledge is acquired. For example, the results of a proposed multicenter collaborative clinical trial to evaluate initial medical vs surgical treatment of primary open-angle glaucoma might change prevailing practice patterns markedly. Therefore, the indications discussed in this chapter are intended to serve as guidelines only and must not be used to regiment patient care decisions.

BIBLIOGRAPHY

Grant WM, Burke JF Jr: Why do some people go blind from glaucoma? *Ophthalmology* 1982; 89:991–998.

Harris LS, Galin MA: Effect on ocular pigmentation on hypotensive response to pilocarpine. *Am J Ophthalmol* 1971;72:923–925.

Primary Open-Angle Glaucoma [Preferred Practice Pattern]. San Francisco: American Academy of Ophthalmology; 1989.

Quality of Ophthalmic Care [Preferred Practice Pattern]. San Francisco: American Academy of Ophthalmology, 1988.

Commentary

E. Michael Van Buskirk, MD

Dr Mills makes some excellent recommendations in defining the patient with glaucoma. In the quest for lower intraocular pressure, it is easy to lose sight of the primary goal of glaucoma therapy: to maintain the optic nerve and the visual field. The glaucoma therapist must refrain from rapidly advancing therapy to an intolerable or unacceptable level in the absence of optic disc findings. Ocular hypertensive patients who fail to respond to tolerable medical therapy may choose simply to be watched, as long as they can cooperate with ocular and visual field examinations. As Dr Mills rightly points out, the approach to maximal medical therapy has become much more complex with the introduction of new medications. Studies comparing beta blockers show that only about 20% of patients exhibit a significant change in intraocular pressure when switched from one beta blocker to another.

The cholinesterase inhibitors should be used with caution if filtration surgery is contemplated because they cause chronic conjunctival and episcleral inflammation, vascular hyperemia, and iris edema. These conditions increase intraoperative bleeding, making the iris more difficult to prolapse, and increase postoperative inflammation. Therefore, I prefer to discontinue cholinesterase inhibitors 2 to 4 weeks prior to surgery. Thus, unless I anticipate a significant drop in intraocular pressure that has a good chance of obviating the need for the surgery, I rarely use cholinesterase inhibitors. An aphakic eye with a poor prognosis for filtration, however, would be a suitable candidate for cholinesterase inhibitors.

CHAPTER 4

Basic Trabeculectomy: Surgical Technique

E. Michael Van Buskirk, MD

Paying meticulous attention to general principles of technique during filtration surgery will permit a higher overall success rate and will allow the surgeon to filter successfully in cases that otherwise would fail. In general, everything possible to minimize the stimulation of fibroblast proliferation should be done. The cutting, spreading, and tearing of tissue should be kept to a minimum. In addition, the surgeon should strive to keep the incisions linear, rather than multilaminate, to maintain as small and localized incisional scars as possible. It is much better to make a definitive linear incision through both conjunctiva and sclera than to make multiple frayed-edged tentative cuts. Furthermore, the tissue should be manipulated as little as possible and the conjunctiva kept moist.

4-1

INITIAL CONJUNCTIVAL INCISION

For the limbus-based trabeculectomy, the initial incision through the conjunctiva should be placed approximately 9 mm posterior to the limbus. The trabeculectomy should be displaced from the center to the superonasal quadrant, leaving the superotemporal quadrant for possible subsequent filtration or cataract surgery.

A bridle suture is usually necessary for a limbus-based trabeculectomy because the conjunctival incision needs to be placed about 9 mm posterior to the limbus (Figure 4-1). The bridle suture should be placed more posteriorly than for typical eye surgery, at least 9 mm behind the limbus.

The initial incision through conjunctiva is exceedingly important. Except for the paracentesis, this is the only step of the procedure for which toothed forceps are indicated. A substantial bite of conjunctiva and underlying Tenon's capsule should be grasped with 3-mm toothed forceps and tented up sufficiently for a small incision to be made through both layers down to

the level of the episclera, 9 mm posterior to the limbus. This can usually be
achieved with a single snip through both
layers using blunt-tipped micro Westcott
scissors. (Sharp-tipped forceps and scissors
should be avoided to minimize inadvertently cutting or traumatizing tissues.)
Looking through the conjunctival incision,
the surgeon can see a small hole through
Tenon's capsule.

After the initial incision, both blades of
the scissors may be inserted into this small
incision to the space beneath Tenon's capsule. The scissors blades are then rotated
to a plane perpendicular to the globe and
slightly separated to lift the conjunctival/
Tenon's capsular flap away from the underlying episclera in both directions. One
blade is then removed and the incision
should be extended to cover about 2 clock
hours just temporal to the vertical meridian nasally (Figure 4-2). When cutting
over the insertion of the superior rectus
muscle, the surgeon should lift the scissors blade toward him so that he can see
the blade through the conjunctival flap to
be sure he has not incorporated any muscle fibers into the incision. The anterior
lip of the wound should then be grasped
on the Tenon's capsule side with fine, ser-
rated, curved, blunt forceps such as the
Gill or Chandler forceps. The flap should
be retracted toward the cornea and lifted
away from the globe. Broad bands of connective tissue adhesions between the underlying episclera and the surface of the
flap will be observed. These can be gently
lysed under direct visualization with scissors held flat to the sclera (Figure 4-3).
Reflection of the flap should then be advanced to the limbal area.

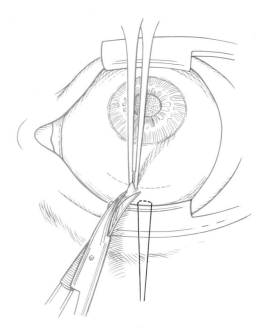

Figure 4-1 *The initial incision through conjunctiva and Tenon's capsule.*

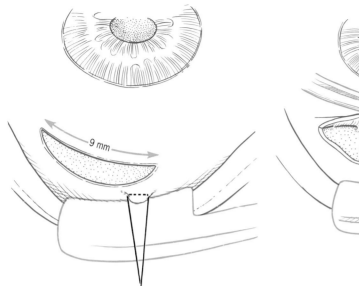

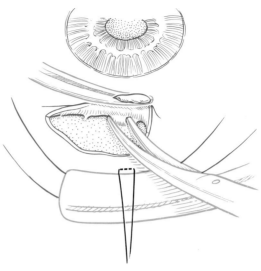

Figure 4-2 *Completion of the conjunctival/Tenon's capsular incision 9 mm posterior to the limbus.*

Figure 4-3 *Anterior dissection of the conjunctival/ Tenon's capsular flap, with excision of Tenon's episcleral fibrous adhesions.*

A small amount of bleeding may be observed from the underlying episcleral vessels. This will usually stop spontaneously and can be managed during the dissection with gentle balanced salt irrigation. Persistent bleeding vessels should be individually cauterized using a bipolar cautery. Controlled cutting of tissue under direct visualization allows the surgeon to avoid the larger vessels such as branches of the anterior ciliary arteries.

The Tenon's capsular insertion will be encountered just at the posterior portion of the surgical limbus. The conjunctiva needs to be reflected anterior to this insertion. The tight adhesions in this area can be lysed with a blunt-tipped small blade, such as the No. 64 Beaver blade, held perpendicular to the surface of the globe

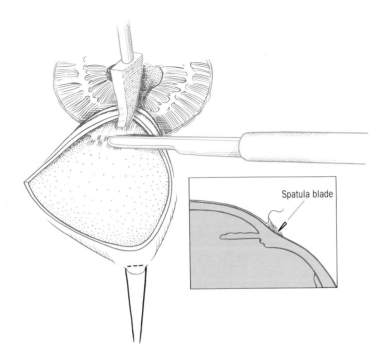

Figure 4-4 *Clearing the limbal reflection of Tenon's capsular adhesions with a spatula blade.*

Spatula blade

parallel to the limbus, advancing the blade forward toward the limbus. This "bulldozing" motion, done gently, will advance the flap well into the surgical blue zone, but special care must be taken to avoid perforating the flap (Figure 4-4). This blue zone reflection of conjunctiva should extend approximately 5 mm in width from the vertical meridian nasally.

4-2

PARACENTESIS

Before the split-thickness scleral flap is prepared, a limbal paracentesis should be made into the anterior chamber. This self-sealing wound permits access to the anterior chamber after the filtration fistula is

made. The paracentesis wound should be placed near the limbus in the horizontal meridian temporally. I prefer a disposable Wheeler-type knife such as the No. 5100 Beaver blade. The conjunctival flap should be replaced to its normal anatomic position. The medial rectus muscle should be grasped through the conjunctiva with toothed fixation forceps. The eye should be retracted nasally with the medial rectus muscle to achieve stability. At the same time, with the other hand, the surgeon should place the tip of the Wheeler knife against the limbus, just superior to the horizontal axis in the temporal limbus and aimed toward the 6-o'clock position (Figure 4-5). The blade should be gently, but firmly advanced through the cornea into

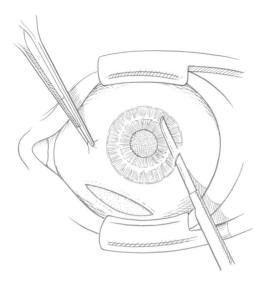

Figure 4-5 *Paracentesis with fixation on the medial rectus muscle.*

the anterior chamber and passed to the full thickness of the blade. This will allow a flat, beveled incision that will be self-sealing and will not require suturing. The blade should enter obliquely to keep the blade over the iris to avoid lens injury. When the blade has advanced to its full width, it should be withdrawn quickly and definitively. This process can often be done without losing any aqueous humor.

4-3

SPLIT-THICKNESS SCLERAL FLAP

A small amount of cautery should then be applied to the limbal area to achieve hemostasis and to prepare for the subsequent preparation of the split-thickness scleral flap. I prefer a trapezoidal trabeculectomy flap, although it can be triangular, square, round, or arch-shaped. I prefer a flap half the scleral thickness, 4 mm in width at the base, 2.5 mm in height, and 2.5 mm in width at the apex (Figure 4-6). The bipolar cautery is used to outline gently an area of these dimensions. The site of the split-thickness scleral flap should be free of all vessels. An ultrasharp mini blade such as the No. 7511 Beaver should then be used to outline the trabeculectomy flap by cutting through 50% of the scleral thickness, creating a trapezoid of the dimensions given above. The incision should be made definitively, without multiple tentative strokes. This will achieve a sharp-edged flap that will lie neatly in its scleral bed at the conclusion of the procedure.

The edge of the scleral flap should then be grasped with Hoskins forceps and gently retracted. A spatula type of blade, such as the No. 6400 Beaver or the No.

681.28 Grieshaber, should be used to split the sclera at the 50% depth. The trabeculectomy flap is then gently separated from the underlying sclera by using a side-to-side motion of the spatula blade (Figure 4-7). When the blade enters a lamellar plane within the sclera, there is little resistance to side-to-side motion.

As the flap is retracted, the underlying bed will be noted to have a white color similar to that of the surrounding sclera, slightly grayer because of the underlying uvea. If the color is quite gray, the flap is too thick and the bed too thin. As the flap is retracted forward, a moderately definitive white line beyond which lies a more grayish blue area is encountered. This white line is the anterior extent of the sclera and approximately overlies the scleral spur, or the posterior extent of the trabecular meshwork. The grayish blue zone anterior to the white line is the oblique junction between the cornea and the sclera and overlies the trabecular meshwork. Approximately 1 mm farther forward, the bluish gray area gives way to a more translucent, nearly transparent zone of clear cornea. This junction corresponds approximately to Schwalbe's line. When clear cornea is encountered, the flap is dissected sufficiently far forward.

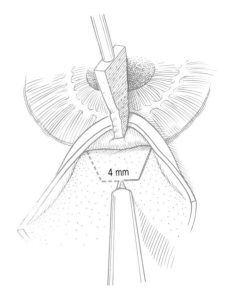

Figure 4-6 *Preparation of a split-thickness scleral trabeculectomy flap 4 mm in width at the base, 2.5 mm at the apex, and 2.5 mm in height.*

4-4

LIMBAL FISTULA

Next, the fistula into the anterior chamber should be prepared. This can be done with one of two methods. I prefer to make an ab externo incision parallel to the limbus, just anterior to Schwalbe's line in the most peripheral portion of clear cor-

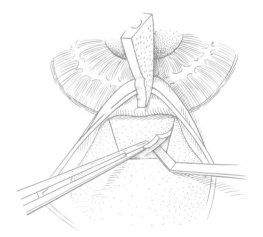

Figure 4-7 *Dissection of the scleral flap from the scleral bed with a spatula blade.*

A

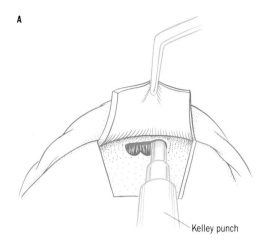

Kelley punch

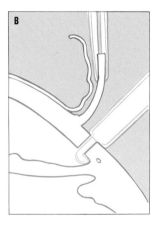

B

Figure 4-8 *Reflection of the scleral trabeculectomy flap, showing limbal landmarks overlying (A) the scleral spur and (B) Schwalbe's line. Preparation of the transscleral fistula with the Kelley punch.*

nea. A mini sharp blade such as the No. 7511 Beaver can be used to create an incision approximately 2 mm in length. It needs to be just long enough to admit the 1-mm tip of the Kelley Descemet's membrane punch, about 2 to 2.5 mm. Again, the incision should be definitive to be sure that it is through and through.

The nondominant hand may then be used to retract the scleral flap over the cornea. The dominant hand should hold the Kelley Descemet's membrane punch and gently insert the tip into the ab externo incision. The shoulder of the tip should rest just under the posterior lip of the wound and be lifted toward the surgeon to avoid pressing on any intraocular structures (Figure 4-8). The punch can then take a bite from the posterior lip of the wound, creating a small semicircular incision. One or two additional bites should be removed from the posterior lip to create a fistula approximately 0.5 to 1 mm in height and 1.5 to 2 mm in width.

An alternative method of creating the fistula is to excise a rectangular block of trabecular meshwork with knife and fine scissors, such as the Vannas scissors. In this technique, two small vertical cuts are made, each approximately 1 mm from the lateral extreme of the scleral bed starting just anterior to Schwalbe's line and extending posteriorly to about the level of the scleral spur, or about 1 mm. Vannas scissors are then inserted into one of these incisions, and the inner blade extended toward the opposite incision. The blade should be extended approximately at the level of Schwalbe's line, just at clear cornea. This will create a flap 1 × 2 mm hinged at approximately the level of the scleral spur. This flap should be retracted toward the surgeon, with the assistant retracting the scleral flap. This trabecular flap can then be amputated with Vannas scissors. The disadvantage of this technique is that the surgeon is more dependent on the assistant to retract the scleral flap during excision of the block.

4-5

IRIDECTOMY

With either technique, the surgeon should allow the iris to prolapse into the fistula. If the fistula is through and through, the iris invariably does prolapse, unless it is rigid and fibrotic as in rubeosis, chronic uveitis, or following long-term cholinesterase inhibitor therapy. When the iris prolapses into the fistula, it should be grasped with nontoothed forceps such as the Pierce-Hoskins and gently retracted. The Barraquer iridectomy scissors should then be held parallel to the limbus and the iridectomy completed (Figure 4-9). The iridectomy should be wide enough to extend from one side of the fistula to the other. It is better for the iridectomy to be too wide than too small. If possible, the surgeon should avoid having to reach into the eye to enlarge the iridectomy because of the risk of lens injury.

The iris will usually reposition spontaneously. If it does not, the trabeculectomy flap should be gently laid over the fistula and the fistula gently compressed through the trabeculectomy flap with the heel of a muscle hook. This will usually disengage the iris from the edge of the fistula. The iridectomy should be visible through the clear cornea, and the pupil should be round.

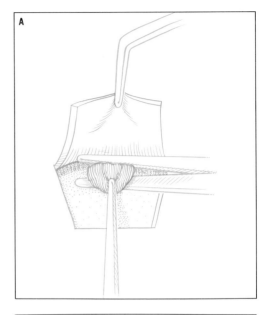

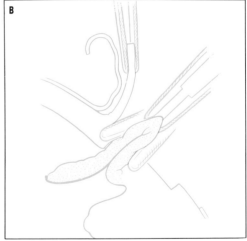

Figure 4-9 *Peripheral iridectomy. (A) The surgeon's view, showing the scissors blade parallel to the limbus. (B) Cross-sectional view.*

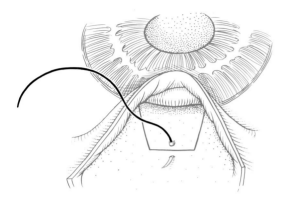

Figure 4-10 *Closure of the scleral flap.*

SCLERAL FLAP CLOSURE

The surgeon is now ready to close the scleral trabeculectomy flap. The flap should be gently laid in its normal anatomic position (Figure 4-10). I prefer to leave the flap quite loose at this stage because many failures result from too tight a closure of the scleral flap, obviating the planned translimbal fistula. A single 10-0 nylon suture is placed in the middle of the apical edge and tied loosely. The suture ends are cut even with the knot, and the knot gently rotated into the scleral channel to prevent the suture tips from eroding the conjunctiva. A blunt-tipped balanced salt cannula can be gently placed under the scleral flap to the anterior chamber, irrigating away any blood or tissue particles.

CONJUNCTIVAL FLAP CLOSURE

The conjunctival/Tenon's capsular flap should then be repositioned to the normal anatomic position. In most cases, the anterior chamber will be formed at this stage but the eye will be very soft. I close the conjunctival/Tenon's capsular flap with a running horizontal mattress suture (Figure 4-11). I prefer an 8-0 collagen chromic suture because it is soft, absorbable, and has a minimal inflammatory response. Other sutures such as 10-0 nylon are equally well tolerated, but nonabsorbable sutures persist and can be disconcerting to the patient. Whenever antimetabolite therapy is

A

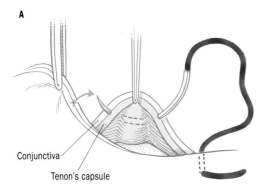

Conjunctiva

Tenon's capsule

B

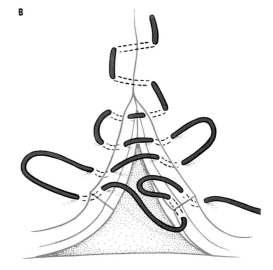

given, a nonabsorbable suture, such as 10-0 nylon, should be used.

The suture is tied to one apex of the wound. The running horizontal mattress technique is performed by grasping the curved needle with the needle holder near the distal end of the needle but on the flat portion. The needle should be held parallel to the wound and within the wound near its apex. Nontoothed forceps such as the Chandler should gently grasp one lip of the wound and pass the conjunctiva over the needle to bring the tip of the needle out on a conjunctival surface. Next, the conjunctiva is grasped again on the same side and again passed over the needle, bringing the needle out on the Tenon's capsule side. The opposite lip of the wound is grasped and the process repeated, feeding the conjunctiva onto the needle and bringing the needle tip out on the conjunctival side to bring the tip out on the Tenon's capsule side. This makes a horizontal mattress loop and

C

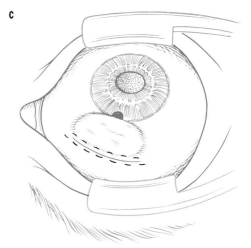

Figure 4-11 *Conjunctival closure with the horizontal mattress suture. (A) The surgeon's view, showing the loops through conjunctiva and Tenon's capsule. (B) Lateral view, showing occasional loops through Tenon's capsule. (C) Finished closure with a distended bleb.*

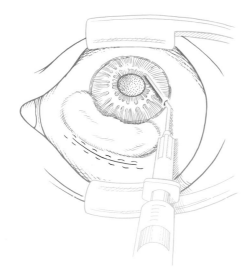

Figure 4-12 *Deepening the anterior chamber and testing wound integrity with a 30-gauge cannula through the paracentesis.*

slightly inverts the edge of the wound. Very small bites should be taken. Multiple bites may then be passed onto the needle (without moving the needle) to close approximately one third of the incision. About every fourth bite, the surgeon should reach under the posterior lip of conjunctiva to grasp the cut edge of Tenon's capsule and feed it onto the needle as well. This will serve to anchor the conjunctival wound posteriorly and prevent it from migrating anteriorly.

The needle will become rather loaded with loops of conjunctiva when about one third of the wound is closed. At this point, the tip of the needle should be grasped and pulled through the conjunctiva onto the underlying suture. The process is repeated to completely close the wound. A knot should then be placed at the distal apex. By this point, the conjunctival bleb has usually formed spontaneously. If the anterior chamber is less than normal depth, it should be deepened just slightly greater than normal depth through the previously placed paracentesis wound, using a 30-gauge cannula on a syringe filled with a balanced salt solution (Figure 4-12).

4-8

CONCLUSION OF THE SURGERY

At the conclusion of the surgery, 1% atropine drops and a mild antibiotic ointment such as polymyxin B sulfate are placed in the palpebral fissure, and the eye is dressed with a dry sterile patch and a Fox shield.

4-9

SUMMARY

For successful trabeculectomy surgery, everything possible should be done to maintain an open translimbal fistula and a functional filtration bleb. The surgeon should proceed definitively, without unduly manipulating the tissues. The conjunctival incision should be placed 9 mm posterior to the limbus, and the conjunctival flap dissected under direct visualization with a minimum of manipulation. A paracentesis provides an access route to the anterior chamber for deepening the chamber and testing the wound at the conclusion of the surgery. A split-thickness scleral flap with smooth edges and plane of dissection should be dissected to the most anterior extreme of the corneal–scleral limbus at the most peripheral extreme of clear cornea. The anterior edge of the fistula should coincide with the junction of the cornea and the anterior extent of the limbus. The iris should be allowed to prolapse to permit an adequate iridectomy without introducing instruments into the anterior chamber. The scleral flap should not be sutured too tightly, but the conjunctival wound should be fluid-tight.

Minimal manipulation of the tissues, definitive surgical technique, and careful attention to surgical anatomy increase the likelihood that a successful filtration bleb will form.

BIBLIOGRAPHY

Lewis RA, Phelps CD: Trabeculectomy v thermosclerostomy: a five-year follow-up. *Arch Ophthalmol* 1984;102:533–536.

Watson PG: Surgery of the glaucomas. *Br J Ophthalmol* 1972;56:299–305.

Commentary

Robert N. Weinreb, MD

As Dr Van Buskirk mentions, attention to technical details should improve the chance of surgical success. The chapter has outlined general principles designed to minimize trauma and bleeding. My surgical approach is similar, but a few maneuvers are different:

1. Before surgery, I pass a traction suture of 6-0 polyglactin 910 (Vicryl) through the peripheral cornea in the superonasal quadrant. The globe is then gently rotated and the suture clamped inferiorly. In comparison to the bridle suture described in the chapter, I find this approach has less chance of hemorrhage and better exposure.

2. Bleeding vessels in episcleral, Tenon's capsular, or conjunctival tissue are meticulously cauterized with fine bipolar cautery. The goal is to achieve a bloodless field. Avoiding blood in the surgical field may minimize fibroblast proliferation and undesirable scar formation.

3. I employ a triangular flap that is 4 mm on each side and hinged at the limbus through one-half thickness of the sclera. I place the paracentesis tract after dissecting the scleral flap, as it is easier to dissect sclera with a pressurized globe. A 10-0 nylon suture is used to reapproximate the apex of the scleral flap.

4. Closure of Tenon's capsular and conjunctival tissue is an important step in trabeculectomy. To ensure a fluid-tight wound closure, I close these tissues in two separate layers. First, I use a continuous 8-0 Vicryl suture to close Tenon's capsule. Second, I use another 8-0 Vicryl suture to close conjunctiva. The anterior chamber is re-formed through the paracentesis tract to ensure that the incision is fluid-tight. Interrupted sutures are added until this is achieved.

5. Minimizing inflammation may best be achieved with subconjunctival injection of methylprednisolone (0.5 cc SoluMedrol) in an inferior quadrant, in addition to postoperative topical glucocorticoids. With a 30-gauge needle, the incidence of subconjunctival hemorrhage is negligible.

Commentary

Richard A. Lewis, MD

My technique for a trabeculectomy is similar to that described in this chapter. In eyes that have undergone previous surgery, it is important to localize mobile conjunctiva. This can best be performed by using a cotton-tipped applicator to search for areas of scarring. Gentle exploration with the cotton-tipped applicator will provide important information that will aid in access to the limbal area through a limbus-based conjunctival flap. The limbal dissection is extremely important and should be carefully performed. I prefer the Gill knife, a blunt blade that provides immobilization of tissue without tearing. It must be emphasized that careful localization of the limbus is critical to successful entry into the anterior chamber. In addition, good hemostasis is essential to provide adequate visualization.

In regard to the scleral flap, my personal preference is a triangle with a half-thickness scleral flap. The sclerostomy should be completed so that there is no question of a clear-cut opening with an enlarged iridectomy underneath it. I close the scleral flap with a single 8-0 polyglactin 910 (Vicryl) suture. I then use the remainder of the 8-0 Vicryl suture as a running two-layer closure, closing first Tenon's capsule and then conjunctiva with a single knot.

At the conclusion of the surgery, I expect to see a shallow but formed anterior chamber with a well-formed conjunctival bleb. The wound must be fluid-tight at the conclusion of the surgery. If there is any question, irrigation through the paracentesis site is advisable to deepen the chamber and enlarge the bleb.

CHAPTER 5

Basic Trabeculectomy: Postoperative Care

Richard A. Lewis, MD

The objectives of a trabeculectomy are to create a permanent fistula through the sclera into the subconjunctival space and to lower intraocular pressure. The effort to create a permanent opening is not physiologic, because the normal biologic response to injury is wound healing with formation of a scar. Several factors conspire against establishing a patent fistula and conjunctival filtering bleb in the first few weeks after surgery, including reduced aqueous flow, intraocular inflammation, and wound healing of all incised tissues. The surgeon must be attentive to these factors throughout the postoperative period because the success of filtration surgery depends not only on the technical aspects of the operation but also on close followup, appropriate intervention, and proper postoperative therapy.

5-1

CARE AFTER UNCOMPLICATED TRABECULECTOMY

For an uncomplicated trabeculectomy, the patient is examined frequently—typically, but not exclusively, on postoperative days 1, 4, 8, and 12; then weekly for 3 weeks. If problems are detected, postoperative examinations are more frequent. Patients should be instructed to avoid vigorous activity, straining, and lifting objects weighing more than 10 pounds. However, the other routine activities of daily living may continue.

The patient is treated postoperatively with topical steroids to control inflammation, topical antibiotics to prevent infection, and a long-acting cycloplegic to relax the ciliary body, deepen the anterior chamber of a phakic eye, and dilate the pupil. Some clinicians have advised additional anti-inflammatory measures with supplemental systemic prednisone (20 mg daily) for the first two postoperative weeks. The cycloplegic and antibiotics are discontinued within 2 to 4 weeks, while the topical steroids are continued for approximately 6 weeks or until inflammation in the anterior segment shows signs of clearing. If employed, 5-fluorouracil (5-FU) is also given during the first two postoperative weeks. The description and dosage recommendations of 5-FU are provided in Chapter 10.

One of the dilemmas encountered in the postoperative management of the glaucoma patient who has undergone trabeculectomy is the use of aqueous suppressants (beta blockers and carbonic anhydrase inhibitors) for the unoperated eye. Aqueous flow through the fistula created in the operated eye is important during this time, and systemic absorption of aqueous suppressants may reduce the flow. Thus, aqueous suppressants should be discontinued prior to the surgery and avoided for as long as possible postoperatively.

5-2

SYMPTOMS AFTER TRABECULECTOMY

Common symptoms after trabeculectomy include blurred vision and mild ocular discomfort. Vision is distorted in the early postoperative period because of varying degrees of inflammation, a shifting of the lens–iris diaphragm with shallowing of the anterior chamber, and alterations in the suprachoroidal space because of hypotony-induced effusions. As the intraocular pressure returns to normal physiologic levels above 6 mm Hg, vision gradually returns to preoperative levels. Ocular discomfort

may arise from tissue manipulation during surgery, from the sutures, and from postoperative inflammation of the conjunctiva and anterior segment. However, severe ocular pain is unusual; if present, intraocular infection or a choroidal hemorrhage should be suspected.

5-3

SIGNS AFTER TRABECULECTOMY

In the early postoperative period, the altered physiologic state of the eye results in common signs. Externally, mild conjunctival injection and inflammation are typical near the bleb and site of wound healing. The most common cause of failure in filtration surgery occurs near this site, at the conjunctival–scleral interface. This results from fibrosis and scarring of episcleral tissue. Thus, maintenance of an elevated bleb is important in the early postoperative period. The bleb should be well delineated, and the intraocular pressure less than 10 mm Hg.

In the postoperative period, intraocular pressure is often low for the first 3 to 14 days. With renewed aqueous flow, healing of the conjunctival wound, and restoration of normal ocular function, the intraocular pressure begins to increase. It is not unusual to note transient elevation at 4 to 8 weeks. Gradually, with remodeling of the wound, the pressure returns to the desired end point in the mid-teens.

The appearance of the bleb and the level of intraocular pressure during the initial 7 to 14 days can be a helpful guide to the problems inherent in the postoperative filter (Table 5-1).

5-3-1 Flat Bleb and High Intraocular Pressure

If the bleb is flat and the intraocular pressure is elevated with a deep anterior chamber, gentle ocular massage through the inferior lid with the eye closed should result in noticeable enlargement of the bleb. Ocular massage can be very helpful in the early postoperative period to maintain the flow through the fistula and remove debris that may obstruct the flow and act as a nidus for bleb failure. Ocular massage is performed by gently pressing the eye through the lower lid while having the patient look upward. If massage is unsuccessful in enlarging the bleb and the intraocular pressure remains elevated in the early postoperative period, the surgeon should consider using the argon laser to cut the suture(s) holding the scleral flap. This requires accurate visualization of the suture with a contact lens applied to the conjunctiva. The Hoskins lens is specifically designed for this purpose, although the corner of the Zeiss gonioprism is quite acceptable (Hoskins and Migliazzo 1984).

A failing bleb typically is flat, injected, and associated with elevated intraocular pressure. After the first 3 to 6 weeks, ocular massage is less effective at enlarging the bleb. If an obstruction to outflow is recognized at the inner ostium of the sclerostomy site, such as an isolated membrane or flap of iris, the Nd:YAG laser may be useful. However, if conjunctiva is adherent to the sclera or if episcleral fibroproliferation is present, resuscitative efforts are generally unsuccessful and surgical revision is necessary.

If the bleb is flat, intraocular pressure is elevated, and the anterior chamber is

TABLE 5-1

Bleb Appearance and Intraocular Pressure Related to Outcome

Bleb Appearance	IOP	Condition
Flat	High	Determine chamber depth: If shallow, pupillary block, malignant glaucoma, or choroidal effusion; If deep, occluded fistula or tight flap
Flat	Low	Wound leak or choroidal effusion
Elevated	High	Encapsulated
Elevated	Low	Desired outcome

shallow or flat, the surgeon should consider and differentiate among malignant glaucoma, pupillary block, and choroidal hemorrhage to initiate appropriate therapy. An uncommon complication of filtration surgery, malignant glaucoma is often associated with primary angle-closure glaucoma. Conservative management includes topical cycloplegic for dilation of the pupil and topical steroids. If unsuccessful, Nd:YAG laser surgery directed at the anterior hyaloid or completion of an anterior vitrectomy is necessary (Brown et al 1986).

5-3-2 Flat Bleb and Low Intraocular Pressure

If the bleb is flat and the intraocular pressure is low, the surgeon should check for a conjunctival wound leak. A strip of fluorescein applied to the conjunctival surface (Seidel test) aids in localizing the site of leakage. A conjunctival wound leak is a special concern in filtration surgery. Small wound leaks may be sealed with a pressure patch and topical aqueous suppressants (beta blockers). It is important to develop a fluid-tight wound as quickly as possible to avoid flattening of the bleb and adherence of the conjunctiva to the underlying sclera. More definitive closure of a conjunctival wound leak may require suture closure, compression (with a Simmons tamponade shell, symblepharon ring, or collagen shield), or cyanoacrylate glue (Melamed et al 1986). Suture closure of a wound leak requires meticulous reapproximation of the wound without

enlarging or worsening the tear. A 10-0 nylon with a tapered needle (as used in microvascular surgery) is well suited for this purpose.

5-3-3 Elevated Bleb

A large bleb may result in corneal dellen formation at its base near the limbus, indicative of surface irregularity with consequent corneal drying. This is a transient problem that most often resolves with wound remodeling. Artificial tears, a lubricating ointment, and antibiotics are necessary if corneal epithelium is absent to provide comfort until the dellen have cleared.

A large bleb associated with elevated intraocular pressure after 3 to 4 weeks may be encapsulated (Van Buskirk 1982). An encapsulated bleb ordinarily resolves with subsequent normalization of intraocular pressure and reduction in size of the bleb. If elevated intraocular pressure persists, topical steroids, aqueous suppressants, and digital pressure may be useful in aiding resolution. Rarely is needling or bleb revision necessary.

5-4

ALTERED ANTERIOR AND POSTERIOR SEGMENT

Other postoperative signs involve the anterior and posterior segment. The anterior chamber displays alterations in clarity and depth. Mild aqueous cell and flare is present for the first few days. Occasionally, a small hyphema or scattered red blood cells are also noted. If blood is present in the anterior chamber, the patient should be instructed to sleep with the head elevated to prevent blood from settling in the sclerostomy site. Anterior chamber depth is often noted to be shallow but formed for the first 1 to 2 weeks. This shallowness is due to an anterior shift of the lens–iris diaphragm, which in part is due to effusions in the choroidal space. These effusions resolve with the return of intraocular pressure to normal physiologic levels above 6 mm Hg.

A flat anterior chamber is more serious, resulting in corneal decompensation and cataract formation. The most common source of a flat chamber is a conjunctival wound leak; however, a large choroidal hemorrhage or effusion may also be the cause. Conservative measures should be exercised, although the chamber should not remain flat for more than a week. Management of choroidal hemorrhage is controversial (Ruderman et al 1986). If the patient is comfortable, no clear benefit is derived from draining the effusion, particularly during the early postoperative period because a hemorrhagic choroidal effusion may recur. Drainage is indicated if associated with severe ocular pain or a prolonged flat chamber. A choroidal hemorrhage is best treated by drainage through one or more sclerostomies while simultaneously deepening the anterior chamber with constant infusion through a limbal paracentesis.

5-5

SUMMARY

The postoperative period is characterized by dramatic changes in the anterior and posterior segment. Attention to these changes with appropriate intervention ensures greater long-term success and fewer complications.

BIBLIOGRAPHY

Brown RH, Lynch MG, Tearse JE, et al: Neodymium:YAG vitreous surgery for phakic and pseudophakic malignant glaucoma. *Arch Ophthalmol* 1986;**104**:1464–1466.

Hoskins HD Jr, Migliazzo C: Management of failing filtering blebs with the Argon laser. *Ophthalmic Surg* 1984;**15**:731–733.

Melamed S, Hersh P, Kersten D, et al: The use of glaucoma shell tamponade in leaking filtration blebs. *Ophthalmology* 1986;**93**:839–842.

Ruderman JM, Harbin TS Jr, Campbell DG: Postoperative suprachoroidal hemorrhage following filtration procedures. *Arch Ophthalmol* 1986;**104**:201–205.

Van Buskirk EM: Cysts of Tenon's capsule following filtration surgery. *Am J Ophthalmol* 1982;**94**:522–527.

Commentary

Robert N. Weinreb, MD

Dr Lewis has provided an overview of postoperative care following trabeculectomy. Careful followup during the postoperative period may be more important to ultimate surgical success than are the technical aspects of the procedure. A number of points are worth amplifying:

1. All of my filtration surgery is done on an outpatient basis. Despite oral and written instructions to patients prior to surgery, the postoperative medical regimen can be bewildering. I have found it useful to examine patients and review medications on postoperative days 1 *and* 2.

2. The sine qua non of wound healing is inflammation. Without inflammation, there can be no wound healing. Hence, I believe it essential to inhibit inflammation as completely as possible during the postoperative period. For me, this has been achieved best by using both topical glucocorticoids and a brief (less than 3-week) course of oral glucocorticoids. Diabetic patients are advised to monitor their urine, and the dosage is tapered more rapidly if necessary.

3. Like Dr Lewis, I am reluctant to employ a systemic carbonic anhydrase inhibitor during the postoperative period, although I am unaware of any well-controlled studies indicating that CAIs make a difference. With rare exceptions, I continue topical beta-blocking agents until the night before surgery. Also, I continue using them in the contralateral eye during the postoperative period if indicated.

4. Digital pressure is an essential component of postoperative care. If a filtering bleb becomes shallow or intraocular pressure increases during the postoperative period, I gently press the eye through the lower lid while the patient gazes upward. Often, this massage is done within the first two postoperative weeks. At this time, I instruct the patient in the appropriate technique for self-administering digital pressure. Its use is adjusted according to the clinical response.

PART II

Trabeculectomy Variations

CHAPTER 6

The Fornix-Based Conjunctival Flap

Robert N. Weinreb, MD

Use of the fornix-based conjunctival flap during glaucoma filtration surgery has increased. Comparison of limbus-based and fornix-based conjunctival flaps during trabeculectomy has indicated that the safety and success of these alternative surgical approaches are similar.

6-1

SURGICAL TECHNIQUE

The superonasal or superotemporal quadrant is selected for dissection. The superonasal quadrant is preferable because it preserves temporal tissue for subsequent filtration or cataract surgery. A temporal quadrant sometimes offers better exposure and is preferable if prior surgery has been conducted in the superonasal quadrant.

The conjunctiva is incised at its limbal insertion for a length of approximately 60° (2 clock hours) with sharp scissors and toothless forceps. The insertion of Tenon's capsule is also incised and gently undermined with blunt scissors. The tissue is spread posteriorly over the area in

which the scleral flap is to be dissected (Figure 6-1). As with trabeculectomy using a limbus-based conjunctival flap, several shapes of scleral flaps can be employed. For dissection of the scleral flap, it is necessary to retract Tenon's capsule and conjunctiva. Toothed forceps may fray the edges of conjunctiva or create buttonholes. Hence, toothless forceps should be employed. Also, a Graether collar button or bent cyclodialysis spatula is useful for retraction of this tissue. If exposure is restricted, the surgeon has the choice of either extending the peritomy an additional 30° (1 clock hour) or performing a radial relaxing conjunctival incision at one end of the peritomy. The dissection of the scleral flap and excision of the sclerotrabecular block are the same as with the limbus-based conjunctival flap.

The fornix-based conjunctival flap is closed at both ends using a 9-0 nylon suture (Figure 6-2). The needle is passed through peripheral cornea or episcleral tissue at the edge of the conjunctival peritomy and parallel to the limbus. A second bite is passed through conjunctiva and the edge of Tenon's capsule approximately 2 to 3 mm from the edge. The opposite

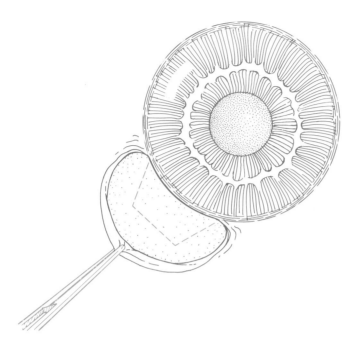

Figure 6-1 *Formation of a fornix-based flap.*

edge of the flap is closed similarly so that the conjunctival margin forms a straight line and slightly indents the superior cornea. The anterior chamber is re-formed through a paracentesis tract, and the integrity of the wound closure tested. The seal should be fluid-tight. Additional interrupted sutures are added as necessary to ensure the integrity of the wound.

6-2

ADVANTAGES

The advantages of a fornix-based conjunctival flap are numerous:

1. Exposure is better than with the limbus-based conjunctival flap. With better visualization, the dissection of the scleral flap anterior to the iris root is facilitated.

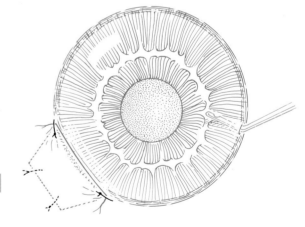

Figure 6-2 *Closure of a fornix-based flap.*

2. Compared to the limbus-based conjunctival flap, the procedure is technically easier and requires less time. Further, the procedure involves less dissection and less bleeding; this is advantageous because there is less likelihood of wound healing being stimulated.

3. A more diffuse bleb may result because there is no posterior scar line to limit the extension of the bleb. The anterior placement of the incision at the limbus is away from the area of filtration. This may limit the extension of the bleb onto the cornea, with fewer cystic anterior blebs overhanging the cornea.

4. Long-term intraocular pressure control is equivalent to that obtained with the limbus-based approach. Also, the number of flat anterior chambers and hypotonic eyes seems comparable.

5. Dissection of the flap is easier when operating in the area of conjunctiva scarred from previous surgery or trauma.

6. After peritomy, conjunctiva is not manipulated until the end of the procedure, when it is reattached. Less manipulation of tissue means fewer conjunctival buttonholes.

7. Wound closure is easier, and less foreign suture material is employed.

8. Because tissue is dissected anteriorly, the possibility of inadvertently incising the edge of a rectus muscle is avoided.

9. The same technique is readily modified for combined trabeculectomy and cataract extraction.

6-3

DISADVANTAGES

Several disadvantages of the fornix-based conjunctival flap are as follows:

1. Inexperience with closure can lead to frequent wound leaks. Achieving fluid-tight closure is more difficult.

2. Surface irregularities in the area of conjunctival wound healing may lead to dellen formation.

3. The fornix-based conjunctival flap is not generally useful with full-thickness procedures.

4. Caution is necessary with the adjunctive use of antimetabolites because final attachment of the flap depends on wound healing.

5. Postoperative wound leaks at the limbus need to be treated by creating additional tension on the free edge of conjunctiva or by placing interrupted sutures on the free edge to the cornea.

6-4

SUMMARY

A fornix-based conjunctival flap provides excellent visualization for trabeculectomy. Fluid-tight wound closure may be difficult to obtain. The fornix-based conjunctival flap is not generally useful with the full-thickness procedure, and caution is advised with the adjunctive use of antimetabolites.

BIBLIOGRAPHY

Shuster JN, Krupin T, Kolker AE, et al: Limbus- vs. fornix-based conjunctival flap in trabeculectomy: a long-term randomized study. *Arch Ophthalmol* 1984;10:361–362.

Traverso CE, Tomey KF, Antonios S: Limbal- vs. fornix-based conjunctival trabeculectomy flaps. *Am J Ophthalmol* 1987;104:28-32.

Commentary

Donald S. Minckler, MD

This chapter clearly summarizes the advantages and disadvantages of the fornix-based conjunctival flap for filtration surgery. Unquestionably, under some circumstances, better exposure and easier, faster surgery can be achieved with this type of flap. Buttonholes in the conjunctival flap are significantly less likely than they might be following dissection of a limbus-based flap in an eye with perilimbal scar tissue or difficult exposure.

The main disadvantage of this technique is that the incidence of wound leak during the first few postoperative days is higher than with the limbus-based flap. The technique is probably not desirable if the cornea is particularly fragile, because the surgery necessarily includes more trauma to the perilimbal corneal epithelium on which healing will depend. An example of the type of patient who would probably not be a good candidate for the fornix-based flap is someone with recurrent herpes epithelial disease.

When using the fornix-based flap for trabeculectomy, I have found it wise to leave the anterior portion of the superficial scleral flap relatively tightly closed to avoid a jet-stream leak from the anterior edge of the scleral dissection. Unfortunately, if a leak along the anterior portion of the conjunctival wound occurs, it almost always requires significant redissection and additional closure of the anterior scleral flap.

CHAPTER 7

The Watson Trabeculectomy

Richard P. Mills, MD

In the standard trabeculectomy, popularized by Cairns and described in Chapter 4, the trabecular block is excised anterior to the scleral spur. An alternate approach to the removal of the scleral block underneath the superficial scleral flap is the Watson variation, in which the trabecular block is excised from the posterior side and includes the scleral spur in the excision. The original idea of the Watson trabeculectomy was to add a cyclodialysis to the filtration procedure. However, a cyclodialysis cleft rarely if ever results, so in practice the Watson variation is similar to the basic trabeculectomy and not at all like a cyclodialysis.

7-1

SURGICAL TECHNIQUE

The initial steps in the operation are the same as in the basic trabeculectomy. A fornix- or limbus-based conjunctival flap is fashioned, followed by a rectangular superficial scleral flap (Figure 7-1), with the lamellar dissection brought well anterior

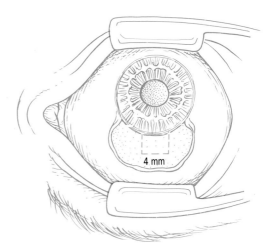

4 mm

Figure 7-1 *A fornix-based conjunctival flap is retracted to allow a superficial scleral flap 4 × 4 mm to be outlined.*

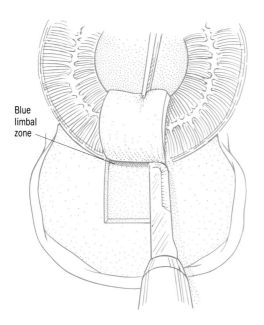

Blue
limbal
zone

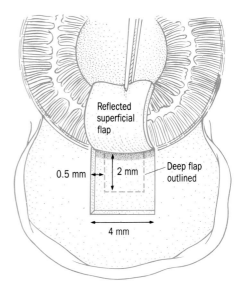

Reflected
superficial
flap

0.5 mm

2 mm

Deep flap
outlined

4 mm

Figure 7-2 *A No. 64 Beaver blade is used to dissect the superficial scleral flap anteriorly beyond the blue limbal zone into clear cornea.*

Figure 7-3 *A deep scleral flap is outlined with a No. 75 Beaver blade.*

into the blue limbal zone until clear cornea is reached and the iris details can be seen through the deep layer of tissue (Figure 7-2). The deep rectangular flap is then outlined with a supersharp No. 75 Beaver blade through the remaining scleral thickness down to the ciliary body (Figure 7-3).

A deep rectangular flap whose sides are 0.5 mm in from the edge of the superficial flap is desired. The posterior extent is 2 mm posterior to the blue limbal zone and is hinged anteriorly. Using a scratching motion with the blade along three sides of the rectangle, the surgeon makes the incision fully through the sclera and will see the dark ciliary body at the bottom of

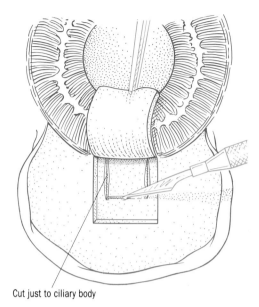

Cut just to ciliary body

Figure 7-4 *The deep flap incisions are deepened until the ciliary body is reached.*

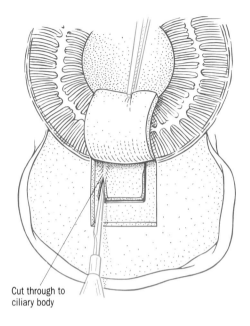

Cut through to
ciliary body

Figure 7-5 *A No. 75 Beaver blade is inserted with the sharp edge pointed upward to complete three sides of the flap to full depth.*

some sections of the incision (Figure 7-4). Scratching down onto the ciliary body may seem risky, but perforating the ciliary body is actually quite difficult because there is a potential space between sclera and ciliary body. Therefore, as the blade comes through, it tends to push the ciliary body away from it rather than penetrating it.

Beginning at a location where the scleral incision is full thickness, the surgeon turns the supersharp No. 75 Beaver blade so the sharp edge is directed up toward the ceiling (Figure 7-5). The point of the blade is inserted the way a letter opener is inserted into an envelope and is advanced along the incision, cutting up

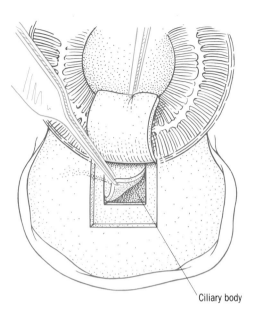

Ciliary body

Figure 7-6 *The deep flap is retracted from the ciliary body, to which it is not adherent.*

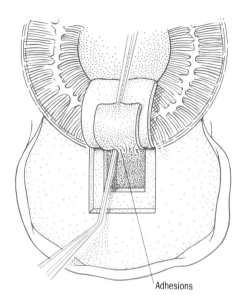

Adhesions

Figure 7-7 *Adhesions are encountered at the insertion of ciliary muscle into the scleral spur. These are divided by sweeping with a blunt instrument such as a cyclodialysis spatula.*

toward the ceiling. This maneuver extends the full-depth scleral incision along all three sides of the rectangle. The deep scleral flap separates easily from the underlying ciliary body because there are no attachments that hold the sclera to the ciliary body behind the scleral spur (Figure 7-6).

As the deep scleral flap peels forward toward the limbus, there is a firm adhesion where the ciliary muscle inserts into the scleral spur. It is so firmly adherent that it is necessary to use a blunt instrument such as a cyclodialysis spatula to tease the insertion away from the sclera (Figure 7-7). Using short strokes directed

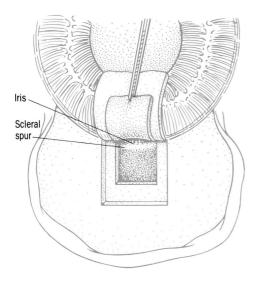

Iris
Scleral spur

Figure 7-8 *After the adhesions are freed, iris, scleral spur, and ciliary body are distinguished by their different textures and colors. The deep scleral flap can then be excised by cutting across the anterior margin with Vannas scissors.*

against the scleral flap at the posterior edge of the insertion, the surgeon can see the ciliary muscle gradually fall away from the sclera. As the muscle drops back, a narrow demarcation line (the previous insertion of the ciliary muscle) divides the dark-brown ciliary body posteriorly from the anterior fine, lacy trabeculation of the iris. The deep flap is then excised by cutting across the anterior edge, which should be in clear cornea (Figure 7-8).

The anatomy is easy to identify, because the scleral spur is such a clear demarcation line. Thus, an iridectomy can be made basal under direct observation without inadvertently removing a piece of ciliary body. Because the anatomy is so apparent, it prevents the "double-cut" iridectomy—a hazard of the standard trabeculectomy, in which a tag of uveal tissue is observed in the depths of the wound after the iridectomy. On attempted excision, it becomes clear that the tag was actually a ciliary process, and brisk bleeding or presentation of vitreous into the wound results.

7-2

ADVANTAGES

Specific clinical situations exist in which the Watson technique has special advantages. For example, in a patient with secondary glaucoma and peripheral anterior synechiae (PAS) or one with neovascular glaucoma, the fibrous PAS may extend far anteriorly onto the cornea. With the standard trabeculectomy, it is difficult to know how far anterior to carry the dissection to ensure that the incision is clear of the PAS. With the Watson technique, the dissection begins posteriorly and the PAS can be separated under direct view as the dissection proceeds forward, continuing anteriorly until no further iridocorneal adhesions are encountered and the aqueous flows freely through the fistula. With some patients, it may be necessary to temporarily abandon the deep flap dissection and extend the superficial flap a bit more anteriorly to allow enough room for the deep flap to clear the PAS. Other clinical circumstances in which the enhanced anatomic visibility of the Watson variation is desirable include sclerocornea and microphthalmos, where anterior limbal landmarks may be obscure, and when training beginning glaucoma surgeons.

7-3

RESULTS

The only published series directly comparing the Cairns and Watson trabeculectomy techniques demonstrated very similar results (Table 7-1). The series emanated from Addenbrooke's Hospital in Cambridge, England, where both Watson and Cairns used their respective techniques. In this series, the control of intraocular pressure without medication was achieved in about 80% of the patients, who were unselected for seriousness of the glaucoma and whose visual acuity was about the same. The complications were fairly similar as well (Table 7-2). Hyphema did not seem to be more common with the Watson technique, as might be expected.

TABLE 7-1

Results Following Trabeculectomy: Followup Greater Than 1 Year

Variable	Anterior (Conventional) Trabeculectomy	Posterior (Watson) Trabeculectomy
Total eyes	255	197
Control of IOP without medication	83%	82%
Visual acuity		
Better	6%	11%
Same	87%	80%
Worse	7%	9%

Source: Reprinted with permission from Watson PG, Grierson I: Early trabeculectomy in the treatment of chronic open-angle glaucoma in relation to histological changes. In: Zimmerman TJ, Monica ML, eds: Controversies in Glaucoma. Int Ophthalmol Clin 1984;24:13–32.

TABLE 7-2

Complications Following Trabeculectomy

Variable	Anterior (Conventional) Trabeculectomy	Posterior (Watson) Trabeculectomy
Total eyes	255	197
Flat anterior chamber with choroidal detachments	9%	10%
Shallow anterior chamber	16%	16%
Hypopyon	3%	2%
Hyphema	27%	28%
Cystic blebs	30%	25%

Source: Reprinted with permission from Watson PG, Grierson I: Early trabeculectomy in the treatment of chronic open-angle glaucoma in relation to histological changes. In: Zimmerman TJ, Monica ML, eds: Controversies in Glaucoma. Int Ophthalmol Clin 1984;24:13–32.

7-4

SUMMARY

The Watson variation is a valid alternative to a standard trabeculectomy. The posterior dissection adds little time or complexity to the procedure and produces essentially equivalent results. The Watson trabeculectomy is a reasonable surgical choice especially when limbal anatomy is obscure or when anterior PAS are present.

BIBLIOGRAPHY

Watson PG: Trabeculectomy: a modified ab externo technique. *Ann Ophthalmol* 1970;2: 199–205.

Watson PG, Barnett F: Effectiveness of trabeculectomy in glaucoma. *Am J Ophthalmol* 1975;79:831–845.

Watson PG, Grierson I: Early trabeculectomy in the treatment of chronic open-angle glaucoma in relation to histological changes. In: Zimmerman TJ, Monica ML, eds: *Controversies in Glaucoma. Int Ophthalmol Clin* 1984;24: 13–32.

Commentary

Donald S. Minckler, MD

As indicated in this chapter, the Watson technique may be especially helpful in that the anatomic landmarks are more clearly defined during filtration surgery in eyes with significant peripheral anterior synechiae or angle distortion related to previous surgery or injury.

In comparing the Cairns and Watson techniques, I wonder if the latter technique is more likely to weaken the eye wall, with a tendency for the ciliary body to prolapse into the fistula. There would appear to be relatively less support of the ciliary body by the sclera. I also suspect a high risk of postoperative bleeding and more postoperative inflammation with the Watson technique.

CHAPTER 8

Full-Thickness Filtration Surgery

Richard A. Lewis, MD

Historically, the earliest filtration operation for glaucoma was the full-thickness procedure. Numerous modifications have been made over the years, but three variations continue to be utilized: the posterior lip sclerectomy, the thermal sclerostomy (or Scheie technique), and the trephination procedure. Recently, various laser devices have been described that perform ab interno or ab externo full-thickness sclerostomies. The goal in each of these procedures is to create an unguarded full-thickness fistula through the sclera to the conjunctiva.

8-1

ADVANTAGES AND DISADVANTAGES

The principal advantage of a full-thickness procedure over a trabeculectomy is lower intraocular pressure. In a 5-year prospective study comparing the two techniques, the average postoperative intraocular pressure was lower after a thermal sclerostomy than after a trabeculectomy (Lewis and Phelps 1984). Consequently, the full-thickness operation is the procedure of choice for patients with low-tension glaucoma and for those with a high risk of failure such as a previously failed trabeculectomy. The full-thickness procedure is also recommended for patients in whom scleral dissection is difficult because of a thin or scarred sclera, but is contraindicated in the presence of limbal scarring.

The creation of an unguarded full-thickness fistula through sclera implies less control of intraocular pressure and greater risk of complications in the early postoperative period (Lewis and Phelps 1984). Complications include hypotony, flat anterior chamber, and choroidal effusion or hemorrhage. In the late postoperative period, the risk of thin blebs and cataract formation is greater.

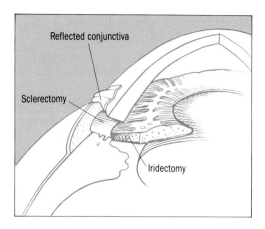

Figure 8-1 *Full-thickness surgery.*

BASIC SURGICAL TECHNIQUE

All full-thickness procedures require careful limbal dissection, sclerectomy, iridectomy, and meticulous conjunctival closure (Figure 8-1). A limbus-based flap is preferred to achieve a fluid-tight wound. Dissection of the conjunctiva should start 6 to 8 mm behind the limbus. Good hemostasis is important to aid visualization as the limbus is approached. Careful blunt dissection is used to clearly delineate the limbal area. A buttonhole of the conjunctiva is especially worrisome with the full-thickness procedure, particularly if it occurs near the limbus. A preplaced paracentesis tract is recommended prior to the sclerostomy to allow access to the anterior chamber at the completion of the surgery—to deepen the chamber, confirm patency of the sclerostomy, and aid in the formation of a conjunctival bleb. Tenon's capsule and conjunctiva are closed in separate layers, and the wound is carefully checked for leakage at the completion of surgery.

POSTERIOR LIP SCLERECTOMY

The posterior lip sclerectomy is performed with a limbus-based flap (Figure 8-2A). The procedure requires an incision 3 to 4 mm through the limbus. The scleral incision should be as anterior on the limbus as possible without creating a conjunctival tear. The anterior incision will allow greater exposure of posterior sclera, to grasp the posterior lip and avoid injury to the lens and other intraocular structures.

A

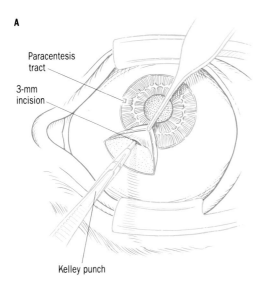

Paracentesis
tract

3-mm
incision

Kelley punch

B

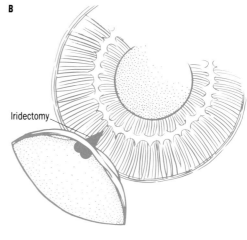

Iridectomy

The sclerectomy is best accomplished with a scleral punch, taking two or three overlapping bites of the posterior lip to obtain a 3-mm opening. It is important to ensure that a full thickness of sclera has been excised, not limited to the more superficial lamellae. Various scleral punch instruments have been used over the years, such as the Kelley, Holth, Walser, or Gass. The Kelley Descemet's punch provides greater control of the tissue and is easier to use. Gentle pressure on the posterior wound will allow prolapse of the iris for the iridectomy (Figure 8-2B).

Figure 8-2 *Posterior lip sclerectomy. (A) A Kelley punch is used to create a 3-mm incision. (B) An iridectomy is performed after the posterior lip sclerectomy.*

8-4

THERMAL SCLEROSTOMY

The thermal sclerostomy (or Scheie procedure) is performed with a limbus-based flap and a partial-thickness incision at the midlimbus of approximately 4 to 6 mm. Then, the surgeon alternates between

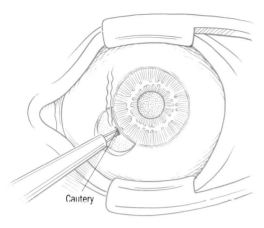

Figure 8-3 *Thermal sclerostomy, or Scheie procedure.*

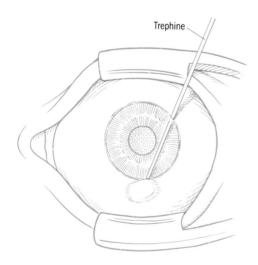

Figure 8-4 *Trephination procedure, in which the sclerectomy is performed with an automated trephine.*

widening the incision with bipolar cautery at both sides of the wound to produce shrinkage and deepening the incision with a blade dissection until entry into the anterior chamber is achieved (Figure 8-3). Care is taken to avoid creating a beveled incision because the sloping margins are more likely to become obstructed, resulting in reduced aqueous flow through the filter. Caution is advised during entry into the eye to avoid lens injury, which is more common with this procedure. A peripheral iridectomy is performed and the conjunctiva is closed.

8-5

TREPHINATION PROCEDURE

The trephination procedure is performed with a limbus-based flap. Of the three, this is the most difficult to perform and the most likely to lead to complications. A 1-mm trephine is applied to the anterior part of the limbus as far anterior as possible. The trephine is carefully depressed and rotated until entry into the anterior chamber is achieved. The sclerectomy excision is completed with scissors.

This procedure is seldom used because there are less control of the tissue during trephination and a greater chance of lens injury. However, a variation of this technique (Brown et al 1987) uses a trabecuphine, an automated trephine with the capacity for simultaneous infusion and cutting (Figure 8-4). This device makes it possible to perform a full-thickness ab interno filtration operation from within the anterior chamber and eliminates the need for a conjunctival incision overlying the fistula.

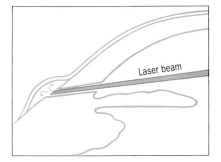

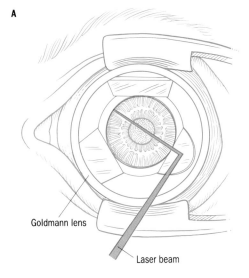

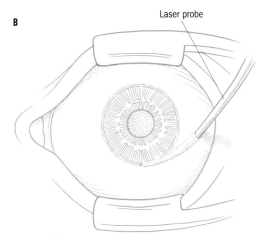

8-6

LASER SCLEROSTOMY

The laser sclerostomy offers promise in the treatment of glaucoma. The principal advantage will be the creation of an ab interno (Figure 8-5A) or ab externo (Figure 8-5B) fistula tract with minimal or no manipulation of the conjunctiva. Various approaches have been described using the Q-switched Nd:YAG, excimer, pulsed dye, and fiberoptic laser techniques with contact and noncontact probes.

8-7

SUMMARY

Full-thickness filtration surgery remains a useful technique, with greater lowering of intraocular pressure than after trabeculectomy. However, short-term complications (including hypotony, flat anterior chamber, and choroidal effusion or hemorrhage) and long-term complications (especially early cataract formation and thinner blebs) are more common.

Figure 8-5 *Laser sclerostomy. (A) Ab interno approach: a laser beam is internally directed into the angle using a contact lens. (B) Ab externo approach: a fiberoptic laser probe is passed through the subconjunctival space and placed contiguous with the area of sclera to be ablated.*

BIBLIOGRAPHY

Brown RH, Denham DB, Bruner WE, et al: Internal sclerectomy for glaucoma filtering surgery with an automated trephine. *Arch Ophthalmol* 1987;105:133–136.

Lewis RA, Phelps CD: Trabeculectomy v thermosclerostomy: a five-year follow-up. *Arch Ophthalmol* 1984;102:533–536.

Commentary

Richard P. Mills, MD

As Dr Lewis has indicated, lower intraocular pressure may be achieved following full-thickness surgery than after a guarded sclerostomy such as trabeculectomy. Full-thickness surgery is not only the procedure of choice for patients with low-tension glaucoma; it may also be advised for patients with high-tension glaucoma who have demonstrated continued deterioration in field and disc with intraocular pressure consistently in the mid-teens. Target pressures of 10 mm Hg and below, for example, may be achieved with full-thickness surgery, but seldom with trabeculectomy.

However, there are good reasons why trabeculectomy has supplanted full-thickness surgery as the standard glaucoma operation. Full-thickness surgery has a higher complication and reoperation rate. A flat anterior chamber with very low intraocular pressure on postoperative day 1 is expected with full-thickness surgery, but is unusual in trabeculectomy. The anterior chamber may re-form in response to cycloplegia or tamponade (pressure patch or tamponade shell) or spontaneously with time. Failure of the anterior chamber to re-form by day 7, requiring surgical drainage of choroidal fluid and re-formation of the anterior chamber, occurs in 20% to 40% of full-thickness operations. In fact, if obtaining operating room time is difficult, the surgeon might provisionally schedule the drainage and re-formation procedure for a week after the original surgery, and cancel the reservation if the chamber re-forms spontaneously. Certainly, patients must be made aware of the likelihood of reoperation so they will not be alarmed if it becomes necessary.

CHAPTER 9

Combined Cataract Extraction and Trabeculectomy

Richard P. Mills, MD

Combining cataract surgery and glaucoma surgery is not a new idea—to do in one operation what would otherwise require two. Until quite recently, however, the combined procedure was not a popular option among ophthalmic surgeons. This is understandable because the classical surgical teachings were at cross-purposes with respect to flat chambers in the two procedures. In full-thickness glaucoma surgery such as trephination, posterior lip sclerectomy, and thermal sclerostomy, a flat chamber was commonplace. If the anterior chamber was not flat or at least sufficiently shallow on postoperative day 1, the prognosis for success of the operation was not favorable. By contrast, in cataract surgery, measures were taken to prevent the anterior chamber from becoming flat.

Before microsurgery and the fine, sharp needles currently available, achieving good wound closure was difficult. A flat anterior chamber usually meant a wound leak and the risk of infection or iris prolapse. Later, when intraocular lenses became available, they were predominantly of iris plane design: medallion lenses,

Copeland lenses, 4-loop Binkhorst lenses. A flat anterior chamber was a disaster, producing irreparable damage to the corneal endothelium. So combining the glaucoma operation with cataract extraction was not deemed to be a good idea.

But now, surgical techniques have changed and the issue of combined procedures is being revisited. With guarded filtration operations utilizing a superficial scleral flap such as trabeculectomy, a flat chamber is an unusual event. Even in the event of a flat chamber, posterior chamber intraocular lenses are less likely to contact the endothelium because of the full thickness of iris between the implant and the cornea.

INDICATIONS

Combined surgery is indicated for a patient with glaucoma and cataract whose pressure is uncontrolled or marginally controlled on maximum tolerable medical management and whose cataract is visually significant or is likely to become so in the near future. The patient should have a significant lens opacity to justify the cataract extraction; likewise, the patient should have a glaucomatous disc or field damage before adding the trabeculectomy.

COMBINED PROCEDURE VS TWO-STAGE SURGERY

The advantages of combining cataract and glaucoma surgery are obvious. The patient incurs less risk and less expense with one operation instead of two. Visual rehabilitation is probably more rapid than with a two-stage procedure. Some evidence indicates that the combined procedure may not be complicated by postoperative spikes in intraocular pressure as frequently as with cataract surgery alone. Because postoperative pressure spikes are more dramatic and more frequent in patients whose outflow is compromised to begin with (patients with glaucoma), avoiding such complications is highly desirable.

The alternative to combining glaucoma and cataract surgery is a two-stage procedure. If the cataract is removed as the first stage in a patient who also needs filtration surgery, the intraocular pressure is not likely to be controlled postoperatively any better than it was preoperatively. This is in contrast to the finding in nonglaucomatous or early glaucomatous eyes, in which cataract extraction frequently normalizes the intraocular pressure (Savage et al 1985). The level of intraocular pressure after the cataract operation in a glaucoma patient is unpredictable. In fact, postoperative pressure control may be worse than it was prior to cataract surgery. Yet some time must be allotted for the eye to quiet down before filtration surgery can be done successfully. Control of pressure during this period is often difficult, particularly if the patient was on maximum medical management preoperatively.

After a cataract operation, the conjunctiva seals down firmly at the limbus, making conjunctival flap dissection during later filtration surgery more tedious if a superior site is chosen. Operating in this area of scarred conjunctiva may predispose to recurrent scarring and failure of the filter. Accordingly, many surgeons place the filtration fistula away from the area of the cataract wound with its scarred conjunctiva. Often, that implies an inferior location, which is an awkward place to operate.

If the cataract is extracted as the first stage, vision recovers quickly but becomes blurred again during the postoperative phase of the second-stage glaucoma procedure, prolonging visual rehabilitation. Finally, the success rate of filtration surgery in a pseudophakic eye is probably less than that in a phakic eye, though probably better than in an aphakic eye (Heuer et al 1984).

In the other variant of the two-stage procedure, the filtration operation is done as the first stage. While the filter matures, which may take 3 months or longer, the cataract may worsen. In patients with only one sighted eye, that delay may be unacceptable.

The cataract extraction should be placed away from the filtration bleb. If the surgery violates an established bleb, fibrosis will be stimulated and the bleb will likely fail. That means the cataract incision must be placed either through clear cornea superiorly or through the limbus temporally or nasally, away from the bleb. Clear corneal incisions may make nucleus expression more difficult and may result in large postoperative astigmatism. A limbal incision, if there is a pre-existing superonasal bleb, would start at the 12-o'clock position and run temporally 4 or more clock hours. That is an awkward incision location for most surgeons and traverses the limbus at its narrowest point (3- or 9-o'clock position). Moreover, cataract surgery in the presence of a functioning filtration bleb causes the bleb to fail about 30% of the time after the cataract surgery, requiring another glaucoma surgery.

glasses in patients with glaucomatous visual field loss simply magnify the scotomas. Contact lenses in patients with filtration blebs carry the risk of endophthalmitis, to a greater degree with large soft lenses than with small rigid ones. An iris-supported intraocular lens is contraindicated if a filter is performed because if the chamber becomes shallow postoperatively, the lens will contact the cornea. An anterior chamber lens in a glaucoma patient may further compromise the angle and further impair aqueous outflow. However, if during cataract surgery the posterior capsule is torn, an anterior vitrectomy is required, and the patient expects an intraocular lens, an anterior chamber lens is often chosen. An alternative procedure is to sew a posterior chamber lens into position in the sulcus. One technique uses a single-piece polymethylmethacrylate (PMMA) lens with heat cautery to make the tips of the haptics bulbous so that a 10-0 polypropylene (Prolene) suture tied around the haptic will not slide off the end. A needle is passed through the inferior and superior ciliary sulcus, and the suture is then tied on the superficial sclera or under a small lamellar scleral flap.

| 9-3 |

INTRAOCULAR LENSES

In combined glaucoma and cataract surgery, posterior chamber intraocular lenses are desirable, mainly because other alternatives have serious drawbacks. Aphakic

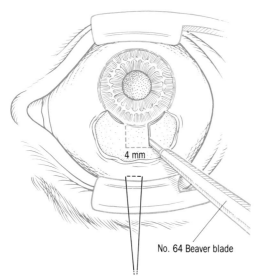

4 mm

No. 64 Beaver blade

Figure 9-1 *A fornix-based conjunctival flap is retracted to allow dissection of a superficial scleral flap 4 x 4 mm.*

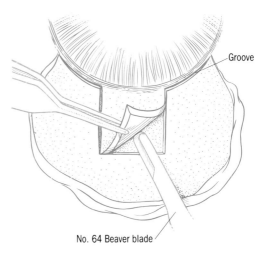

Groove

No. 64 Beaver blade

Figure 9-2 *A No. 64 Beaver blade is used to dissect the superficial scleral flap and create a partial-thickness limbal groove incision across the full width of the cataract incision.*

9-4

SURGICAL TECHNIQUE

The overwhelming consensus is to do the combined procedure using a fornix-based flap because the visibility of the capsulotomy and the cortical cleanup are impaired by a limbus-based flap flopping down over the cornea (Figure 9-1). The superficial scleral flap (rectangular, triangular, or circular) is outlined approximately half the scleral thickness with a No. 64 Beaver blade. The flap is placed either in the center of the cataract wound, for convenience, or at either end of it. A partial-thickness groove is extended along the limbus on either side of the superficial scleral flap (Figure 9-2). It is important to

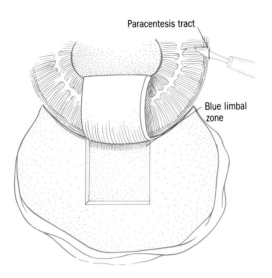

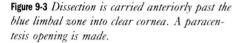

Figure 9-3 *Dissection is carried anteriorly past the blue limbal zone into clear cornea. A paracentesis opening is made.*

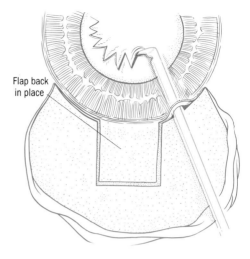

Figure 9-4 *A 1-mm incision is made at one side of the trabeculectomy flap to admit the cystotome, and an anterior capsulotomy is done.*

dissect the lamellar scleral flap in a firm eye, which facilitates the maintenance of consistent depth in the dissection. A paracentesis should be done after the flap dissection, also while the eye is firm (Figure 9-3). If the paracentesis is done first and a little aqueous leaks out softening the eye, dissection of the superficial flap is more difficult.

The superficial scleral flap is dissected well forward into clear cornea, forward of the blue zone where the cataract incision is placed. Adjacent to the anterior corner of the superficial scleral flap, but in the limbal groove, a stab incision is made into the anterior chamber and a standard capsulotomy is performed (Figure 9-4). Then, with the scleral flap reflected, a super-

Figure 9-5 *A No. 75 Beaver blade is used to enter the chamber across the most anterior part of the dissection in clear cornea. This incision is continued with corneoscleral scissors to the full width of the groove. The lens nucleus is expressed.*

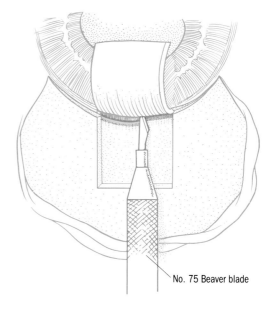

No. 75 Beaver blade

Figure 9-6 *Two temporary sutures are placed to hold the wound closed, and the remaining lens cortex is aspirated.*

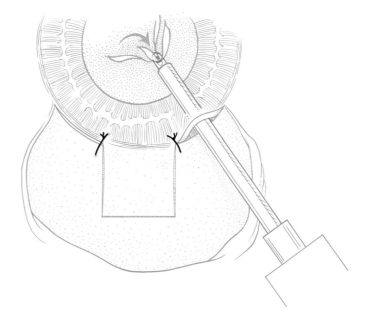

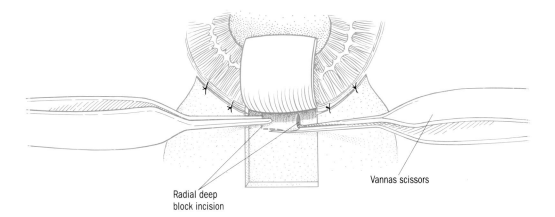

Radial deep
block incision

Vannas scissors

sharp No. 75 Beaver blade is used to enter the anterior chamber across the width
of the lamellar dissection (Figure 9-5). In
the center of the flap, the anterior chamber entry incision is quite far anterior, but
curves back along the edges to meet up
with the groove at the limbus. Corneoscleral scissors extend the cataract incision
to adequate width (between 10 and 11
mm, depending on lens nucleus size).
The lens nucleus and cortex are removed
in the usual fashion (Figure 9-6), followed
by implantation of the posterior chamber
intraocular lens. The portion of the
wound outside the scleral flap is closed
with 10-0 nylon. Finally, the deep block
of corneoscleral tissue is excised with Vannas scissors or a Kelley Descemet's punch,
thus completing the trabeculectomy (Figure 9-7). By waiting until the end to excise the deep block of tissue, the surgeon
preserves enough wound integrity to allow
maintenance of the anterior chamber during irrigation and aspiration.

An iridectomy across the width of the
trabeculectomy opening is performed
(Figure 9-8), and the scleral flap is tacked

Figure 9-7 *The cataract incision away from the trabeculectomy site is closed. Two radial incisions
are made from the anterior deep incision line
back to the scleral spur. The deep block is then
excised with Vannas scissors.*

A

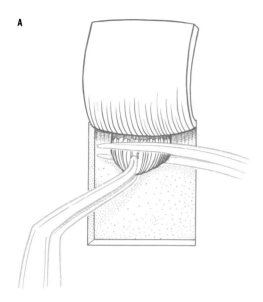

B

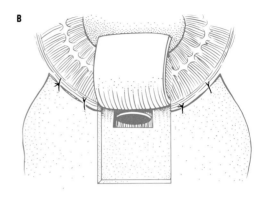

Figure 9-8 *(A) An iridectomy is performed.
(B) After the iridectomy, ciliary processes can
sometimes be seen and should not be cut.*

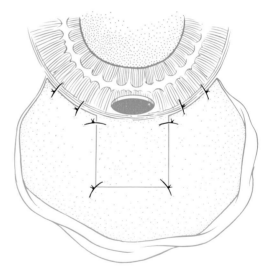

Figure 9-9 *The superficial scleral flap is then sutured at the corners and near the limbus, where
leaks are most likely to occur.*

down with 10-0 nylon. It is important to place a suture to stabilize the anterior corner of the flap where it meets the limbus to avoid leakage under the edge of the fornix-based conjunctival flap (Figure 9-9). Finally, the conjunctiva is sutured at the corners under some tension so that good apposition at the limbus is achieved, with a small amount of overlap of the conjunctival edge on the cornea (Figure 9-10).

Many glaucoma patients have been on long-term miotics, so that the pupil does not dilate adequately for nucleus expression during extracapsular cataract extraction or for safe phacoemulsification. A properly dilated pupil is the best insurance against zonular dehiscence (especially in a glaucoma patient who has pseudoexfoliation) and posterior capsule rupture. If the adequacy of dilation is questionable, it is wisest to improve the dilation surgically. Just before capsulotomy, Vannas scissors can be introduced through the wound and small sphincterotomies performed at the 4-, 6-, and 8-o'clock positions. A few small sphincterotomies usually work as well as one large one and do not require suturing at the end of the surgery. If the pupil still is not large enough, then a peripheral iridectomy can be made superiorly and converted into a sector iridectomy.

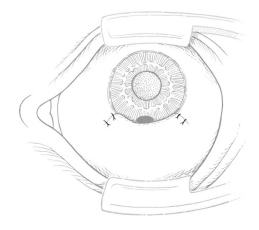

Figure 9-10 *The conjunctiva is closed under some tension with slight limbal overlap.*

9-5

RESULTS OF COMBINED PROCEDURE

The literature is replete with statistics about combined glaucoma and cataract surgery. Most of the early reports concerned intracapsular cataract surgery, and are only of historical interest. Combined intracapsular extraction with trabeculectomy, subscleral posterior lip sclerectomy, and other glaucoma procedures resulted in success rates of 40% to 60% (Galin et al 1985). When authors commented on the quality of the resulting blebs, they usually said the blebs were flat or nonexistent.

Of more interest to current practice are series of extracapsular extractions combined with trabeculectomy (Percival 1985, Simmons et al 1987, McCartney et al 1988, Murchison and Shields 1989). Higher rates of pressure control were reported than in the intracapsular groups. One series of 108 cases achieved a 92% success rate of intraocular pressure control. The inclusion criteria limited entry to the study to patients with glaucoma who were either under good control or under marginal control on medications. This represents a less serious kind of glaucoma than some of the other reported series, which may account for the high rate of success.

9-6

POSTOPERATIVE CARE

Postoperatively, the surgeon should be alert for early intraocular pressure rises and wound leaks. In a fornix-based flap, a wound leak appears under the edge of the conjunctival flap and flows in the gutter between the conjunctiva and the cornea. While ocular compression (massage) is a useful maneuver when a standard trabeculectomy bleb is failing in the early post-

operative period, it should be used with great caution in combined procedures. The reason is that the incidence of optic capture by the pupil in combined procedures is high in the first place and is made even worse by massage before the implant is well seated in position. If the patient compresses and distorts the eye, the intraocular lens may decenter and rotate a bit, capturing the pupil. Once that happens, it is usually permanent. The result is unsightly and may lead to chronic inflammation or optical aberrations.

Patients who have had combined procedures need to know that it is going to take them longer to see well than their friends or relatives who had only their cataract removed. Even after a standard cataract operation, visual rehabilitation is more prolonged in glaucoma patients, and this is especially true after combined surgery.

9-7

SUMMARY

Combining cataract extraction (with posterior chamber lens implantation) and trabeculectomy is a desirable alternative to two separate operations in selected patients with uncontrolled or marginally controlled glaucoma and significant lens opacity. Even if long-term filtration is not established, the combined procedure usually blunts the postoperative intraocular pressure spike that often accompanies cataract extraction alone.

BIBLIOGRAPHY

Galin MA, Obstbaum SA, Asano Y, et al: Trabeculectomy, cataract extraction, and intraocular lens implantation. *Trans Ophthalmol Soc UK* 1985;104:570–573.

Heuer DK, Gressel MG, Parrish RK II, et al: Trabeculectomy in aphakic eyes. *Ophthalmology* 1984;91:1045–1051.

McCartney DL, Memmen JE, Stark WJ, et al: The efficacy and safety of combined trabeculectomy, cataract extraction and intraocular lens implantation. *Ophthalmology* 1988;95:754–763.

Murchison JF Jr, Shields MB: An evaluation of three surgical approaches for coexisting cataract and glaucoma. *Ophthalmic Surg* 1989;20:393–398.

Percival SPB: Glaucoma triple procedure of extracapsular cataract extraction, posterior chamber lens implantation, and trabeculectomy. *Br J Ophthalmol* 1985;69:99–102.

Savage JA, Thomas JV, Belcher CD, et al: Extracapsular cataract extraction and posterior chamber lens implantation in glaucomatous eyes. *Ophthalmology* 1985;92:1506–1516.

Simmons ST, Litoff D, Nichols DA, et al: Extracapsular cataract extraction and posterior chamber lens implantation combined with trabeculectomy in patients with glaucoma. *Am J Ophthalmol* 1987;104:465–470.

Commentary

Richard A. Lewis, MD

A variety of different techniques for performing combined cataract and trabeculectomy procedures have been proposed over the years, and no one way is absolutely correct for all surgeons. The increasing popularity of phacoemulsification with small intraocular lens implants may offer some advantages. In particular, a smaller corneoscleral incision may reduce subsequent fibrosis and scarring of the trabeculectomy. Despite this advantage, it is more important for surgeons to use the technique they are most comfortable with to minimize complications. This is particularly true when considering phacoemulsification for glaucomatous eyes. These eyes often have miotic pupils, with or without posterior synechiae, that cannot be dilated. Manipulation of the iris, which may be more rigid, is associated with greater release of pigment. These circumstances increase the risk of phacoemulsification and necessitate greater planning throughout the surgery. When in doubt, it is important to proceed with a sector iridectomy. This can be closed at the completion of the procedure using a 10-0 polypropylene (Prolene) or left open for greater visualization of the fundus. Further, there may be a greater risk of iris capture of the intraocular lens and subluxation. Thus, it is important to complete this surgery with the confidence that the lens is well positioned and secured in the posterior chamber. A large intraocular lens implant, at least 7 mm, is recommended to prevent iris capture.

Postoperative dilation of the pupil is avoided for the first 6 to 8 weeks. Normally, these patients require greater followup. The eye with combined cataract extraction and trabeculectomy requires close postoperative care to monitor complications and intraocular pressure. Gentle ocular massage can be carefully used to enhance formation of the fistula and enlargement of a bleb.

Commentary

E. Michael Van Buskirk, MD

The issue of combining filtration surgery with cataract extraction is more rife with controversy and variations in technique than many other areas of glaucoma surgery. Like many aspects of cataract surgery, there is more opinion than consensus. As Dr Mills states, combined procedures have been used for many years, although prior to 1970 combined cyclodialysis with cataract surgery was perhaps the more popular approach. I do believe the more recent use of trabeculectomy for the glaucoma portion and extracapsular extraction with posterior chamber intraocular lens implantation for the cataract portion has improved the success rate of combined surgery, but well-controlled studies are difficult to conduct. Most glaucoma surgeons, however, would undoubtedly agree that the predicted success rate of filtration when combined with cataract extraction is somewhat less than when filtration is performed alone. The controversy concerns whether or not the filtration success with the combined procedure is comparable to that with a two-stage approach, and good data are not at hand. However, when cataract extraction becomes necessary after a filtration procedure has been performed, I believe that the filtration bleb should be well established, preferably with the patient not taking pressure-lowering medications. Further, the longer the period of time between filtration and cataract surgery, the greater the chance for preservation of the bleb. I insist on at least 6 months before cataract extraction after trabeculectomy. If it is not feasible to wait 6 months, then I proceed with combined surgery.

The small-incision approach to cataract surgery seems relevant to this discussion. The small-incision cataract extraction with phacoemulsification is particularly suitable for the glaucoma patient because it violates a smaller area of the limbus, allowing extraction well away from a functional bleb with a two-stage approach. It also permits phacoemulsification entirely under a trabeculectomy flap, with only minimal modification to insert an intraocular lens at the end of the surgery. This allows the glaucoma surgeon to modify the trabeculectomy to permit removal of the lens, rather than forcing the cataract surgeon to modify the cataract operation to permit filtration.

Glaucoma patients on long-term therapy often have small pupils, which can make phacoemulsification hazardous, especially for the inexperienced surgeon. Therefore, I entirely agree with the need for adequate pupillary dilation. Usually, sufficient dilation can be achieved by pharmacologic and mechanical means. Posterior synechiae can be broken by sweeping under the pupillary margin with a long narrow spatula. Filling the anterior chamber with hyaluronate often distends the pupil over the surface of the lens, dilating it to 5 to 6 mm, which is adequate for phacoemulsification at the iris plane. Only in those patients in whom adequate dilation cannot be obtained do I perform sphincterotomies. I have found bleb failure and postoperative inflammation to be correlated with the amount of intraoperative iris manipulation, particularly sphincterotomies.

I do not regard the limbus-based flap an impediment to a combined procedure. After the aspirating cannula is inserted into the anterior chamber, the limbus-based conjunctival flap can be reflected back over the sclera and the cannula, permitting full visibility of the cornea and anterior chamber.

With any approach, I have found a higher incidence of postoperative inflammation, dimple-like posterior synechiae to the posterior capsule, and iris capture of the edge of the intraocular lens than in cataract surgery without filtration.

Postoperatively, these patients need to be examined more frequently than those having standard cataract surgery or even standard trabeculectomy. After the combined surgery, patients require topical corticosteroids every 2 hours for the first several days and at least four times a day for several months to minimize inflammation.

Because aphakic and pseudophakic eyes seem to have a higher incidence of filtration failure than do phakic eyes, an argument could be made for the use of antifibroproliferative agents such as 5-fluorouracil with the combined procedure, although I have not taken that approach thus far.

CHAPTER 10

Antimetabolites and Filtration Surgery

Robert N. Weinreb, MD

Postoperative subconjunctival injections of 5-fluorouracil (5-FU) are employed to enhance the surgical outcome of glaucomatous eyes with poor prognoses undergoing filtering surgery. This antimetabolite is of value because filtration failure is often due to episcleral fibrocellular proliferation. By inhibiting the enzyme thymidylate synthase, 5-FU blocks deoxyribonucleic acid synthesis and, presumably, inhibits episcleral fibrocellular proliferation.

10-1

PREOPERATIVE CONSIDERATIONS

Adjunctive use of 5-FU is indicated in glaucomatous eyes with poor surgical prognoses, including aphakic eyes, eyes with previous failed filtering procedures, and eyes with neovascular glaucoma. Use of 5-FU with primary filtration surgery that has a good prognosis has been suggested, but is not established. Prior to filtering surgery in neovascular glaucoma, regression of iris neovascularization should be obtained by retinal photocoagulation or retinal cryoablation. In all cases, it is desirable to ameliorate intraocular inflammation by the use of glucocorticoids before undertaking filtering surgery.

Eyes with abnormal lid function, faulty lid apposition, or corneal and conjunctival disease often have corneal epithelial changes during the postoperative period if 5-FU is employed. Thus, a thorough check of lid movement and apposition should be made before surgery. The conjunctival and corneal epithelium, as well as the tear film, should be examined closely. Schirmer tests and rose bengal stain may give additional information. If significant disease is found, the potential risks of using 5-FU should be considered along with the benefits.

SURGICAL TECHNIQUE

The technique for filtering surgery is similar to that in which adjunctive use of 5-FU is not employed. Attention to several steps during the surgical procedure will ensure the best possible outcome:

1. The limbus-based conjunctival flap is the preferred surgical approach because it allows greater security of wound closure.

2. Hemostasis is vigorously maintained during all steps of the procedure.

3. In eyes without prior filtering surgery, the superonasal quadrant is the desired surgical site. In eyes with previous filtering procedures, a site that has not been dissected previously is chosen.

4. A paracentesis incision is made with a sharp knife placed temporally and directed inferiorly toward the 6-o'clock position. This incision is made to facilitate the re-formation of the anterior chamber, inflate the bleb, assess the fluid-tight status of the conjunctival incision closure, wash out blood or debris from the anterior chamber, and assess the resistance of the scleral flap during trabeculectomy.

5. Closing Tenon's capsule and conjunctiva in separate layers may facilitate fluid-tight wound closure at the completion of the procedure. Also, secure closure of Tenon's capsule reduces tension on conjunctiva and may prevent retraction of the wound edges and migration of the suture line. Since inhibition of the healing of the conjunctival and Tenon's capsule incision is not necessarily desirable, a reactive suture such as 8-0 polyglactin 910 (Vicryl) can be used. Alternatively, 10-0 nylon and special microvascular needles are employed by some surgeons.

POSTOPERATIVE CARE

After filtration surgery, patients are given glucocorticoids and assessed for possible antimetabolite therapy:

1. To most effectively ameliorate intraocular and extraocular inflammation, topical glucocorticoids should be administered frequently. Systemic glucocorticoids may be used also for 2 to 3 weeks for maximum anti-inflammatory effect.

2. In eyes with a deep anterior chamber, intact corneal epithelium, and fluid-tight closure, 5.0 or 7.5 mg of 5-FU (0.10 to 0.15 ml; 50 mg/ml) is administered subconjunctivally using a 30-gauge needle on a tuberculin syringe. One drop of topical proparacine 0.5% is used as anesthetic. The injection site selected is posterior to the conjunctival suture line or in a quadrant adjacent to the filtering bleb and at least 8 mm posterior to the limbus. Placing the 5-FU near the site of filtering surgery ensures maximum tissue levels of the antimetabolite for therapeutic effect. Alternatively, some surgeons dilute the 5-FU in sterile saline and administer it 180° from the filtering bleb. Sterile balanced salt solution is used to wash any excess 5-FU from the conjunctival sac and cornea immediately following injection.

3. In general, the patient is assessed for possible antimetabolite injections daily during the first two postoperative weeks. The injection is withheld if there is any sign of conjunctival complication or corneal toxicity.

10-4

COMPLICATIONS

A subconjunctival injection of 5-FU inhibits episcleral fibroblast proliferation nonselectively. All dividing cells are probably affected, including corneal epithelium and conjunctival epithelium. Because 5-FU nonselectively inhibits cell replication, the conjunctival incision may not heal properly and a persistent aqueous humor leak can jeopardize the formation of a filtering bleb during the postoperative period. This risk can be minimized by using a two-layer closure of Tenon's capsule and conjunctiva and ensuring the fluid-tight integrity of the wound at completion. Interrupted sutures can be added until the wound is fluid-tight. The same is true for conjunctival buttonholes. They need to be closed using a microvascular needle so that they are fluid-tight and do not jeopardize the postoperative formation of the filtering bleb.

The most common complications associated with postoperative use of 5-FU are corneal. Mild to moderate corneal changes

include superficial punctate keratitis, filaments, small epithelial defects (less than 1.5 mm in diameter), large sheet-like epithelial defects, edema, and subepithelial scarring. Severe corneal complications include herpetic, bacterial, and fungal ulceration, sterile corneal ulceration and perforation, and keratinized plaque. The most frequent changes seen are superficial punctate keratitis, filaments, and small epithelial defects. These are often noted during the period of active drug administration, although they may arise even after drug administration has been discontinued.

Severe corneal complications often occur in the setting of nonresolving persistent epithelial defects, particularly when topical steroids are being administered. Problems with epithelial healing usually occur within the first few weeks after surgery, although complications such as microbial keratitis sometimes occur several months after surgery.

Corneal changes associated with the use of 5-FU following filtering surgery appear to be dose-dependent. Adjusting the dose of 5-FU according to the clinical response can reduce the incidence of corneal complications. Withholding injection at the time of surgery and even on the first postoperative day, as well as staggering injections over several days, appears to increase corneal tolerance. The placement of a small-volume, high-concentration injection well posterior of the cornea and the use of artificial tears may also be effective in diminishing corneal complications.

Awareness of the early signs of 5-FU corneal toxicity and prompt treatment further reduce complications. Superficial punctate keratitis and filaments appear to be early signs of corneal toxicity. These most likely arise from direct effects of the 5-FU on corneal epithelium with inhibition of epithelial cell division. Their presence may be heralded by a foreign-body sensation. Both superficial punctate keratitis and filaments may occur before an actual epithelial defect. It is important to diligently exclude their presence before giving an injection of 5-FU, because continued drug injection may exacerbate the corneal problem. If these corneal changes are noted, the 5-FU injection is withheld. Despite withholding the subconjunctival injection, these corneas may still worsen. The biologic effect of 5-FU may persist longer than its mere presence would suggest, causing further changes.

If an epithelial defect arises, topical steroids should be discontinued and the eye patched daily until the defect is healed. Patching for several days may be required. Healing of the corneal epithelium may take longer than expected, probably because of persistent biologic activity of the 5-FU. The use of 5-FU is temporarily ceased, and reinstituted only when the epithelium is intact.

10-5

SUMMARY

Many adjunctive therapies have been proposed to increase the success and prevent or reduce the incidence of complications associated with filtering surgery. Postoperative subconjunctival injections of 5-FU have found a place as adjunctive therapy for eyes with otherwise poor prognoses following filtering surgery.

BIBLIOGRAPHY

Fluorouracil Filtering Surgery Study Group: Fluorouracil filtering surgery study one-year follow-up. *Am J Ophthalmol* 1989;108:625–635.

Heuer DK, Parrish RK II, Gressel MG, et al: 5-Fluorouracil and glaucoma filtering surgery, II: a pilot study. *Ophthalmology* 1984;91: 384–394.

Weinreb RN: Adjusting the dose of 5-fluorouracil after filtration surgery to minimize side effects. *Ophthalmology* 1987;94:564–570.

Commentary

Donald S. Minckler, MD

The addition of 5-fluorouracil subconjunctival injections to the postoperative course following trabeculectomy in complicated glaucoma appears to be a major advance. A study supported by the National Eye Institute has clearly demonstrated in a large group of prospectively randomized patients that 5-FU adds significantly to the success rate at 1 year following surgery.

The principal problem with this technique is the logistical difficulty it may create, requiring daily examinations and injections for at least several days following surgery. Additionally, the potential for corneal epithelial damage is significant. As pointed out in the chapter, daily examinations prior to 5-FU injections should detect developing epithelial problems, at which time 5-FU dosage can be adjusted or administration deferred. The most practical way to use this medication is on a "custom" basis, with close monitoring of the patient's response to avoid damaging side effects. Whether 5-FU should be started the day of surgery or 24 hours later is a matter of controversy. Additionally, some controversy exists about the optimum location of the injection sites. Many surgeons prefer to inject 180° away from the filtering bleb.

Commentary

E. Michael Van Buskirk, MD

Dr Weinreb makes excellent points regarding the indications, methodology, and postoperative assessment of a patient undergoing 5-fluorouracil adjunctive therapy. Regarding indications, I would not agree that all patients with previously failed filtering procedures should have 5-FU. The administration of 5-FU is relatively simple and benign, so when indications for its use are in doubt, it probably should be given. The fact is, however, that some filters fail not because of intrinsic wound-healing characteristics of the patient but rather because of extrinsic, improper, technical factors introduced by the surgeon. When these can be identified in a patient who otherwise exhibits no poor prognostic factors, trabeculectomy can be readily performed at a separate site without adjunctive therapy. Revisions of previously failed filters should virtually always be accompanied by 5-FU therapy.

Dr Weinreb's point regarding the importance of wound closure is an important one. Healing of the conjunctival wound may be delayed until after the 5-FU injections have been discontinued. A rapidly absorbable suture such as 8-0 chromic collagen will usually be completely absorbed by 2 weeks, and the wound can dehisce at that time in the presence of 5-FU therapy. I would therefore advocate the use of a nonabsorbable suture such as 10-0 nylon.

The administration of 5-FU is both simple and painless. A cotton pledget, prepared by removing a wisp from a cotton applicator stick, should be saturated with 0.5% proparacaine and placed in the conjunctival sac for 2 minutes. This completely numbs the conjunctiva and allows repeated subconjunctival injection in the most squeamish of patients. The option of administering or withholding 5-FU on a daily basis gives the surgeon maximal ability to titrate the dose.

The conjunctiva can exhibit adverse effects similar to those described for the cornea, including punctate erosion, epithelial defects, and through-and-through holes. The conjunctiva should be observed for white ischemic areas, dimpling, or staining with fluorescein. These are harbingers of conjunctival thinning, leakage, or through-and-through perforation and indicate the need to reduce or withhold the dose.

CHAPTER 11

Implantation of Drainage Devices

George Baerveldt, MD
Donald S. Minckler, MD
Richard P. Mills, MD

For many years, ophthalmologists have attempted to establish artificial aqueous drainage to control intraocular pressure through the use of various implanted devices. Such devices have included horsehair, black silk sutures, platinum, and glass tubes. In 1959, Epstein demonstrated that after implantation, a capillary tube remained patent indefinitely at the anterior chamber end. At the subconjunctival end, a bleb formed initially, but over the ensuing weeks the bleb contracted around the external opening, and the external subconjunctival opening became occluded by a dense fibrous cap.

Molteno devised a large plastic episcleral plate, 13 mm in diameter, which after implantation becomes surrounded by a fibrous capsule that cannot adhere to the smooth plastic surface. Thus, a fluid-filled space is created and maintained by the explant, which acts as a spacer preventing fibrous contraction from obliterating the cavity. The extensive surface area usually allows adequate rates of aqueous percolation through the fibrous capsular wall. As originally described, these large episcleral plates were sutured to the surgical limbus,

extending back to the muscle insertions and connecting to a short tube that protruded into the anterior chamber. This device created huge anterior blebs that frequently caused corneal problems, especially dellen.

A long-tube Molteno implant was then developed, with the same episcleral plate sutured between and posterior to the muscle insertions, creating a large filtering bleb in the equatorial region of the globe. Different plate designs and the inclusion of a one-way pressure-sensitive valve in the tube represent other variations in the successful anterior-chamber-tube-to-episcleral-plate concept for drainage devices.

11-1

PATHOPHYSIOLOGIC PRINCIPLES

All of the various shunt devices utilize identical pathophysiologic principles. Histologic studies in humans and experimental animals have demonstrated that the inner surface of the capsule (filtering bleb) is normally an open meshwork of collagenous tissues without a lining epithelium. Aqueous passes through the capsule by simple passive diffusion and accumulates in the periocular connective tissues (intercellular space). Removal of aqueous from the periocular tissue is by capillaries or lymphatics. Experimental studies have shown no significant resistance across the tube, with identical pressures in the anterior chamber and filtering bleb. It has been suggested that the drainage achieved is proportional to the surface area of the explant. Continual remodeling and thickening of the bleb wall may sometimes result in a relatively impermeable barrier to filtration with clinical failure.

11-2

INDICATIONS

Drainage tubes should be reserved for the most severe cases because the surgical procedure is difficult and many complications can attend their use. Such patients include those in whom conventional trabeculectomy has failed with or without 5-fluorouracil (5-FU) or whose prognosis for trabeculectomy is poor, as in neovascular or active uveitic glaucoma.

Because higher complication rates than in standard trabeculectomy can be expected, implantation of drainage devices should be limited to patients who have inadequate intraocular pressure control on maximum tolerated medical therapy and have undergone numerous ocular surgical procedures, including trabeculectomy, or who fall into a high-risk group of failure with standard trabeculectomy. For example, phakic eyes with glaucoma are selected if they have had two failed filtering surgeries and/or a failed filtering surgery with 5-FU treatments. In aphakic eyes, a single prior failed filter or the presence of other high-risk characteristics is sufficient indication for drainage device implantation. Drainage implants as a primary procedure may be performed on patients with neovascular glaucoma or glaucoma with active uveitis, as primary trabeculectomies even with adjunctive 5-FU have a dismal success rate. Use of drainage implants in the congenital glaucomas depends on the type of congenital glaucoma and the clinical response to goniotomy or trabeculectomy. In all patients, the preservation of some useful residual visual function may justify the hazards and expense of the surgery.

11-3

SURGICAL TECHNIQUE FOR MOLTENO IMPLANTS

Because of the difficulty in precise positioning of the tube within the anterior chamber and the myriad intraoperative and postoperative complications that can occur with deficient technique, drainage implants should be installed only by surgeons thoroughly trained in their use.

Using an operating microscope, the surgeon fashions either a superonasal or a superotemporal limbus- or fornix-based conjunctival flap. The incision for a limbus-based flap should be approximately 6 mm posterior to the limbus. If a single-plate implant is used, the incision is limited to one quadrant, while a 160° incision is required for a double-plate implant. The choice depends on the surface area likely to be required to sustain adequate aqueous drainage. Superior quadrants are usually preferred. However, other factors might direct the surgery inferiorly such as the ability to close conjunctiva over the implants, absence of anteriorly placed peripheral anterior synechiae, which make tube placement difficult, or the presence of intraocular silicone oil.

The conjunctiva and Tenon's capsule are dissected anteriorly to the limbus. Posteriorly, with blunt dissection, Tenon's capsule is lifted from the sclera. The Molteno tube is flushed with a saline solution to ascertain its patency, using a 27-gauge cannula that fits snugly into the tube. The plate is then slipped posteriorly between the sclera and Tenon's capsule so that its anterior edge lies approximately 8 to 10 mm posterior to the limbus. Two nonabsorbable sutures—5-0 or 6-0 polyester (Dacron or Mersilene)—are inserted through the two anterior suture holes on either side of the tube and sutured to the sclera 10 mm posterior to the limbus. If a double-plate implant is selected, the tube connecting the two plates can be passed over the intervening rectus muscle, obviating the difficult step of slipping one plate under the muscle to the adjacent quadrant. To avoid kinking of the tube connecting the two plates, the plates must be placed as far apart as practicable in the adjacent quadrants, and the check ligaments of the intervening rectus muscle must be divided quite far posteriorly.

The tube is cut to the correct length for insertion into the anterior chamber by laying the tube over the limbus onto the cornea. The tube is cut 1 to 2 mm anterior to the limbus with a sharply angled bevel facing anteriorly to facilitate introduction and to allow later Nd:YAG membranotomy of the ostium if necessary. A paracentesis tract is then made into the anterior chamber through clear cornea away from the tube entry site.

If the tube is placed in the anterior chamber and aqueous drainage is not temporarily restricted until a fibrous capsule forms around the plate, severe postoperative hypotony can be expected. A number of methods have been devised to deal with the problem. Molteno originally described the implantation of the device in two separate stages. In stage 1, the plate is installed and the tube is tucked back along the plate and sutured to the episclera. A standard trabeculectomy in a different quadrant may provide pressure control for a few weeks. In stage 2, the tube is released, cut to length, and installed in the anterior chamber.

Alternatively, a temporary absorbable ligature can be tied tightly near the tube–

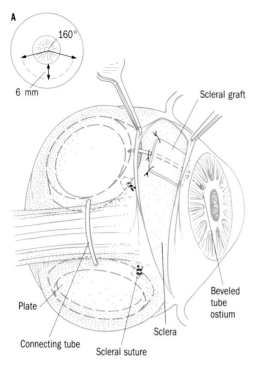

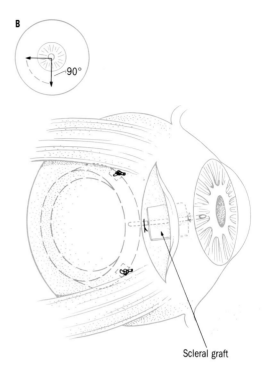

Figure 11-1 *(A) A double-plate Molteno implant in place, with the connecting tube running over the intervening rectus muscle. (B) A single-plate Molteno implant. Donor scleral patch graft covers the tube from the plate to the limbal entry point.*

plate junction to occlude the lumen of the tube. Unfortunately, suture dissolution is unpredictable and a minor reoperation to cut the suture is often necessary (30% to 50% of cases). Slip knots may be used, but may release spontaneously too early or fail to slip on demand. Laser lysis of an occluding suture in the anterior chamber has been advocated, but produces suture debris. Laser energy cannot reliably penetrate conjunctiva and Tenon's capsule to divide tube sutures external to the sclera. A 4-0 chromic "rip cord" can be threaded into the tube, with the other end externalized in the conjunctival cul-de-sac and tacked down using a small-diameter soft suture. The chromic suture swells to occlude the tube lumen and can be pulled free in 7 to 10 days. Care is necessary to avoid breaking the suture when pulling it free, and a small risk of infection is incurred.

A 22- or 23-gauge needle is used to produce an opening in the anterior chamber approximately 0.5 mm posterior to the surgical limbus so that the needle parallels the iris surface. Viscoelastic material may be injected if a deep anterior chamber is desired. The needle is withdrawn, and the Molteno tube is introduced through this opening into the anterior chamber. If the tube is too long, it can be withdrawn and trimmed. The anterior few millimeters of the tube should be covered with a donor scleral graft from an eye bank eye. Adequate elution of the preservative in which the sclera is stored must be accomplished. A strip 4 × 6 mm or larger is cut freehand and cleaned of pigment as much as possible. The strip is applied over the Molteno tube and sutured at the four corners to the sclera with 8-0 polyglactin 910 (Vicryl) sutures. The tube needs to be covered from the limbus to approximately 6 mm posterior to the limbus to minimize later erosion and externalization of the tube (Figure 11-1). Tenon's capsule is closed in a separate layer with a running 8-0 polyglactin suture followed by closure of the conjunctiva. The anterior chamber is re-formed through the paracentesis tract. Subconjunctival injection of antibiotic and steroid is given.

In aphakic vitrectomized eyes, the tube can be placed through the pars plana to lie behind the iris well away from the corneal endothelium. Care needs to be taken that the tube does not catch the residual vitreous skirt and drag it centrally.

11-4

COMPLICATIONS UNIQUE TO DRAINAGE DEVICES

The rate of complication is higher in patients undergoing Molteno implant than in those having a regular trabeculectomy. In part, this is a function of patient selection, because only high-risk patients have drainage devices implanted. But in part, the increased complications result from the difficulty of the surgery and the use of large plastic implants.

Immediate postoperative hypotony with the Molteno implant when it is installed in a single stage has been associated with a high rate of choroidal hemorrhage. With the modifications in technique permitting two-stage operations (two operations or temporary occlusion of the tube), the incidence of choroidal hemorrhage has not been more than that expected with standard filtering surgery in high-risk eyes.

Other complications unique to shunt devices include contact between the tube and the cornea, iris, or lens and erosion of the tube or explant through overlying tissues. Obstruction of the anterior chamber end of the tube may follow bleeding, fibrovascular membrane formation, or migration of the tube into the eye wall. Infection around the tube or explant has been unusual, as has the occurrence of endophthalmitis. Retinal tears or even detachment may follow inadvertent globe perforation during installation of the explants. Muscle imbalance with diplopia has occurred rarely after double-plate installations. A relatively common postoperative "hypertensive phase," often lasting weeks to months, has been observed once the tube is opened. We believe this transient rise in intraocular pressure stems from inflammation triggered by beginning aqueous flow, similar to the encapsulated-bleb phase following trabeculectomy in many patients. As with standard filtering operations, time often effects an improvement in function, presumably as the collagen in the bleb wall remodels to a more permeable configuration.

Supplemental medication is often required following the implant surgery. The majority of patients are controlled on beta blockers alone. Carbonic anhydrase inhibitors produce a further decrease in intraocular pressure. Following a Molteno implant, intraocular pressure responds best to medications that decrease aqueous production. Even if the patient responded dramatically to pilocarpine treatment before implantation, the patient may have minimal decrease in intraocular pressure with pilocarpine afterward. In certain instances, the intraocular pressure can even increase with miotics. Epinephrine and its related compounds are effective in some patients.

11-5

SUMMARY

Drainage devices offer a new surgical method to control intraocular pressure in patients with failed multiple filtering surgical procedures or in patients in the high-risk group for failure of the traditional filtering surgeries. Complication rates are definitely increased in all these patients. Despite the increase in complication rate, the success rate is encouraging.

Further studies need to examine the effect of increasing the size of the equatorial explants to obtain further decrease in intraocular pressure and to investigate whether increasing the filtration area increases the complication rate significantly.

All drainage devices appear to increase the outflow of aqueous from the eye. In patients who fail this type of surgery, cycloablative procedures remain a good alternative for treatment. There is a theoretical advantage of first establishing outflow and then titrating outcome with these cycloablative procedures.

BIBLIOGRAPHY

Hitchings RA, Joseph NH, Sherwood MB, et al: Use of one-piece valved tube and variable surface area explant for glaucoma drainage surgery. *Ophthalmology* 1987;94:1079–1084.

Minckler DS, Heuer DK, Hasty B, et al: Clinical experience with the single-plate Molteno implant in complicated glaucomas. *Ophthalmology* 1988;95:1181–1188.

Molteno ACB: New implant for drainage in glaucoma: clinical trial. *Br J Ophthalmol* 1969;**53**:606–615.

Schocket SS: Investigations of the reasons for success and failure in the anterior shunt-to-the-encircling-band procedure in the treatment of refractory glaucoma. *Trans Am Ophthalmol Soc* 1986;**84**:743–798.

Commentary

Richard A. Lewis, MD

The technique of implanting a Molteno tube is quite varied. I have found it most useful to perform the complete procedure in one session. Using a fornix-based conjunctival flap, I suture the Molteno plate 8 to 10 mm from the limbus with two interrupted 5-0 nylon (Dermalon) sutures. The tube is tied off with a 6-0 polyglactin 910 (Vicryl) suture, which also passes through sclera. The tube is then introduced into the eye through a 23-gauge needle tract. The tube is covered with donor scleral tissue, which is sutured in place with four interrupted 8-0 Vicryl sutures. The conjunctiva is reapproximated to the limbal area with an 8-0 Vicryl suture, ensuring a good, fluid-tight structure.

The most significant postoperative problems following Molteno implant surgery are related to intraocular pressure. When the tube is sutured closed, intraocular pressure postoperatively can be as high as, or higher than, preoperative levels. This necessitates continuation of the preoperative medications and close obser-

vation until the suture is absorbed. An enlarged sclerostomy opening may be helpful to allow for greater drainage in the early postoperative period. However, when there is too much leakage or an open tube, the pressure can be dangerously low, increasing the risk of a choroidal hemorrhage.

It is particularly important that the Molteno tube be well covered with donor sclera. Inserting the tube into the anterior chamber underneath an elongated scleral flap may aid the entry of the tube; however, there may be insufficient protection against erosion of the overlying partial-thickness sclera and conjunctiva. The added thickness of donor sclera is an important aspect in the prevention of this distressing complication. However, caution must be continually exercised because the tube, as well as the implant, is foreign material and is at risk for extrusion and infection.

Commentary

Robert N. Weinreb, MD

I have found few indications for the use of available drainage devices to lower intraocular pressure. In glaucomatous eyes with a poor surgical prognosis undergoing filtering surgery, I employ 5-fluorouracil as adjunctive treatment. I consider the use of a drainage device if 5-fluorouracil is ineffective, and in eyes with congenital or juvenile glaucoma with multiple failed goniotomies or trabeculotomies, eyes with conjunctival scarring several millimeters posterior to the limbus (making the limbus-based flap difficult to dissect), and eyes with marked irregularities of the corneal surface. On occasion, a patient cannot be observed daily because of transportation difficulty or other problems. Drainage devices are sometimes useful in these situations as well. In eyes with inflammation, I have often found subconjunctival injections of 5-fluorouracil with filtering surgery to have a beneficial effect. Several patients requiring long-term glucocorticoid administration to control inflammation have been tapered from steroids after such surgery. I have found that eyes with neovascular glaucoma in which iris neovascularization has not regressed have a poor prognosis regardless of which surgical treatment is employed.

PART III

Complications of Filtration Surgery

CHAPTER 12

Intraoperative and Postoperative Complications

Donald S. Minckler, MD

Glaucoma filtering surgery has always been plagued by relatively high complication rates. Compared to modern cataract surgery, glaucoma surgery continues to be labor-intensive and far more likely to be a difficult experience for patient and physician alike. Major improvements in postoperative management after trabeculectomy have recently included laser suture lysis, removable sutures, and periocular injection of 5-fluorouracil. This chapter concentrates on the most obvious and serious intraoperative and postoperative complications of trabeculectomy.

12-1

PHYSIOLOGY OF FILTRATION BLEBS

The exact mechanisms by which filtering procedures work are presumed to include varying degrees of transconjunctival flow into the tear film and seepage into the periocular intercellular space. The removal of aqueous from subconjunctival spaces is by uptake through capillaries or lymphatic vessels. The goal of the surgical fistula is to bypass the normal outflow apparatus and establish a persistent leak of aqueous into periocular tissues (Katz and Spaeth 1989). Intrascleral filtration, decrease in aqueous production following surgery, planned or unplanned cyclodialysis, and uveoscleral outflow may explain long-term success in the absence of an obvious external bleb. Possibly, transient relief of intraocular pressure by the surgical creation of a fistula and the washing out of pigment or debris promotes repair and improved function of the normal outflow pathways in some patients.

Microcyst formation in the conjunctiva, reflecting transconjunctival fluid movement, is often associated with good bleb function. Filtering bleb boundaries—usually acellular, compressed fibrous tissue—have variable thicknesses and permeability. Clinical observations and histologic studies reveal that functional blebs may have a wide spectrum of internal architecture, including simple, open, fluid-filled cavities and cicatrix formation. The physiologic mechanism of aqueous movement through the bleb wall is probably by simple passive diffusion (Minckler et al 1987). In most cases destined for long-term success, the conjunctival inflammatory reaction is maximal during the first 3 or 4 weeks and has subsided by 6 weeks after surgery.

12-2

EXPECTATIONS AND INFORMED CONSENT

Patients should be informed that the primary goal of filtering surgery is to stabilize intraocular pressure at an acceptable level and prevent further pressure-induced damage to vision. Many patients assume that visual acuity or visual field loss will be improved by filtering surgery. Besides the other more likely complications, patients should be warned that glaucoma surgery has a small risk of further damaging vision. Permanent loss of vision during or after filtering surgery is possible, especially if serious complications ensue. The risk of further vision damage as an immediate consequence of filtering surgery has been variably estimated (5% to 15%) and is probably greatest in patients with the most advanced optic nerve injury, especially in those with split fixation (Katz and Spaeth 1989, Agarwal and Hendeles 1986,

Kolker 1977). One-eyed patients will be especially anxious during the common transient decrease in vision postoperatively. Recovery to the best vision may be prolonged, requiring weeks to many months after completion of surgery in any eye with advanced optic atrophy.

Acceleration of cataract formation is a well-established visual consequence of filtering surgery and should be mentioned during the informed consent.

12-3

FAILURE OF THE PROCEDURE

The most common complication of filtering surgery is failure to achieve stable control of intraocular pressure. Published estimates of success after filtering surgery vary widely (20% to 90%), depending on definitions and especially on length of followup. Failure of both initial and subsequent filtration procedures is most likely during the first few weeks to months following surgery and continues to occur indefinitely at a decreased rate. The average duration of benefit from the first filtering procedure is approximately 5 years. Filtration blebs typically undergo continual, slow remodeling, often with gradual localized or diffuse thinning of the conjunctiva or shrinkage of the bleb boundaries.

The most common cause of bleb failure after trabeculectomy is sealing of the surgical fistula by fibrovascular proliferation at the episcleral surface along the edges of the scleral flap. Experimental studies have suggested that the maximal fibroblastic proliferation around the fistula site occurs between 3 and 7 days postoperatively. Clinically, the most problematic period is between the first and fourth weeks. By 6 weeks, it is usually clear whether or not the procedure will succeed. Failure after full-thickness procedures may also be due to fibrovascular proliferation between the conjunctiva and the episcleral surface. The presence of aqueous between the episclera and the conjunctiva (elevated bleb) with substantial physical separation of the two surfaces probably inhibits bridging by fibroblasts.

During the first few days postoperatively, ocular massage, argon laser rupture of scleral sutures, or release of a removable suture may re-form a flat bleb by re-opening the scleral wound. After suture rupture or removal, the trabeculectomy flap may elevate and fuse with the overlying conjunctival stroma as proof of the ongoing fibrous reaction and contraction along the episcleral surface. Besides sealing of the scleral fistula at its external surface, an established bleb's function may dwindle gradually due to decreasing permeability of its wall (conversion to an encapsulated bleb) or by continual remodeling and obliteration of the filtering cicatrix between the scleral fistula and the undersurface of the conjunctiva. In patients under the age of 50 or patients who have

had previous ocular surgery, especially previous filtering surgery, the chances of success are significantly decreased. Other mechanisms for filtration surgery failure include plugging of the fistula internally by ciliary processes or iris or proliferation of endothelium over the opening. The lens may prolapse into the fistula, or vitreous may extend through a ruptured zonule into the internal opening. During evaluation of a failing filter, gonioscopy is indispensable in clarifying the mechanism involved. Gonioscopy most often reveals a persisting internal opening or cleft, and the block in outflow can be localized to the episcleral surface.

12-4

RETROBULBAR HEMORRHAGE

Retrobulbar hemorrhage as a result of retrobulbar block is often immediately indicated by proptosis or marked tensing of the lids with increased intraocular pressure. The majority of retrobulbar hemorrhages elevate intraocular pressure only transiently, and the elevation will subside rapidly without intervention. With severe hemorrhages in patients with badly damaged optic nerves, rapid relief of the rise in intraocular pressure may require lateral canthotomy to decompress the orbit. Usually, retrobulbar hemorrhage is confirmed by the appearance of blood diffusing to the insertion of Tenon's capsule near the limbus within an hour or two after the event. Retrobulbar hemorrhage should prompt delay of surgery because of the variability of effect on intraocular pressure

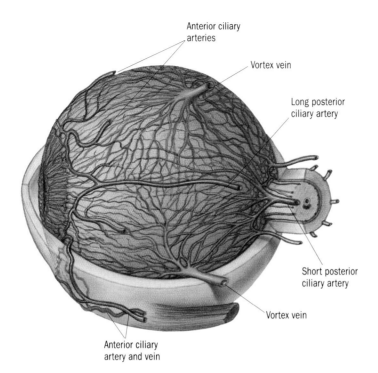

Figure 12-1 *The uveal blood vessels and vortex veins. Hypotony during filtering surgery may impair venous outflow through the vortex veins and cause effusion or hemorrhage in the choroid.*

Modified by permission from Hogan MJ, Alvarado JA, Weddell JE: Choroid. Histology of the Human Eye. Philadelphia: WB Saunders Co; 1971:320–392.

Anterior ciliary arteries

Vortex vein

Long posterior ciliary artery

Short posterior ciliary artery

Vortex vein

Anterior ciliary artery and vein

and the risk of extrusion of intraocular contents or additional intraoperative bleeding. At least a 3-week delay is desirable to permit resolution of blood under Tenon's capsule. If the patient's systemic health permits, general anesthesia is preferable at the next attempt.

12-5

CHOROIDAL HEMORRHAGE

The pathophysiology of choroidal hemorrhage during or after surgery includes ocular hypotony as the principal common denominator. Distortion of the ocular wall during surgery and a number of other risk factors are probably important, including advanced age, arteriosclerosis, previous ocular surgery, certain congenital anomalies, inflammation, and clotting disorders. Ocular hypotony during or after surgery may cause scissoring of the draining vortex veins by scleral collapse and induce choroidal venous congestion with increased risk of choroidal hemorrhage (Figure 12-1). Perpendicularly oriented feeding arterioles may shear, causing arterial choroidal bleeding. Resolved previous choroidal hemorrhage may not increase the risk of choroidal hemorrhage in the same eye at subsequent surgery, but should alert the surgeon to increased risk in the opposite eye with initial surgery.

The risk of intraoperative choroidal hemorrhage is particularly high (around 30%) in patients with nanophthalmos or the Sturge-Weber syndrome. Nanophthalmic eyes have extremely thick sclera and may rapidly develop choroidal effusion or hemorrhage when the eye is opened. Eyes with glaucoma associated with the Sturge-Weber syndrome often contain a choroidal hemangioma, which can undergo rapid expansion or hemorrhage during surgery. Buphthalmic or highly myopic eyes with thin, easily distorted sclera are probably also at increased risk for choroidal hemorrhage during intraocular surgery.

Choroidal hemorrhage during filtering surgery is less likely to be expulsive than during large-incision cataract surgery. The risk of self-limited choroidal hemorrhage during filtering surgery is not known because few surgeons routinely examine the posterior pole at the end of the procedure. Mild to moderately severe intraoperative choroidal hemorrhages that self-tamponade are probably common. The most common time of occurrence of symptomatic choroidal hemorrhage, frequently heralded by a boring pain in the eye, is 24 to 72 hours after filtering surgery (delayed nonexpulsive choroidal hemorrhage).

The signs of intraoperative choroidal hemorrhage include sudden increase in intraocular pressure (unexpected hardness of the eye), the appearance of an expanding choroid in the anterior vitreous cavity, and prolapse or expulsion of intraocular contents. Suspicion of choroidal hemorrhage should prompt immediate attention to controlling the wound to facilitate internal tamponade. Simple compression of the wound for several minutes with intermittent release of ocular compression may effect tamponade, as may completion of scleral flap sutures. Scleral incision over an expanding choroidal mass to vent bleeding externally is seldom effective because the blood quickly loculates and clots. If scleral drainage is attempted, only the scleral wall needs to be opened, as blood is most likely accumulating in the suprachoroidal space immediately deep to the inner scleral surface. Incision into the substance of the choroid itself is likely to aggravate bleeding. The site of entrance should be that ordinarily used to tap choroidal effusions, 3 to 4 mm posterior to the limbus. Gentle exploration along the inner wall of the sclera with an iris sweep may facilitate venting of blood accumulating more posteriorly. Chronic choroidal hemorrhage in eyes examined in the pathology laboratory is almost always maximal at the equator of the globe, although the precise origin of the bleeding is usually not identified. Intravitreal or anterior chamber blood may appear if the choroidal hemorrhage ruptures through Bruch's membrane and the pigment epithelium.

After successful release of blood, the scleral drain site should be left open in case of recurrent hemorrhage. Instillation of fluid, air, or gas into the eye may aid internal tamponade, but must be done with care to avoid inducing extremely high intraocular pressure. Preplacement of scleral fistulas before opening the eye in especially high-risk eyes (nanophthalmos, Sturge-Weber) has been advocated by some as a wise precaution.

12-6

DELAYED CHOROIDAL HEMORRHAGE

Choroidal hemorrhage occurring after wound closure, during the first few days postoperatively, should be treated conservatively. Most delayed choroidal hemorrhages are self-limited and gradually resolve on their own, often without bad effects on the visual outcome. Signs of postoperative choroidal hemorrhage include shallowing of the anterior chamber, a dark-colored expansion of the choroid, and, in the case of rupture into the vitreous, blood in the vitreous cavity or anterior chamber. The principal symptom of choroidal hemorrhage is a boring pain in or around the eye. Many descriptions of choroidal hemorrhage after intraocular surgery indicate that a vigorous Valsalva maneuver (especially straining at stool) may trigger the event. Choroidal effusion probably commonly precedes choroidal hemorrhage. Serous effusion between the retina and the pigment epithelium commonly occurs in eyes with choroidal hemorrhage and may persist even after the hemorrhage has resolved.

Surgical intervention with drainage of choroidal hemorrhage is indicated if pain or intraocular pressure cannot be controlled medically. Choroidal drainage with pars plana vitrectomy should be performed if kissing choroidal hemorrhages persist beyond 1 to 2 weeks, or immediately if surface reaction (gliosis or fibrosis) threatens to weld the inner retinal surfaces together. Ultrasound demonstration of "mobile" blood in the choroid, implying lysis of the clot, has been a favorable finding in my experience, providing a high likelihood of being able to surgically drain persisting choroidal hemorrhage. Pars plana vitrectomy with intravitreal gas instillation to flatten the retina may be indicated. Pars plana vitrectomy after trabeculectomy should be preceded by tight closure of the flap to minimize the extension of infused fluid into the subconjunctival space. In any case, air or gas injected after vitrectomy often escapes through an open filter.

If an unacceptable rise in intraocular pressure occurs immediately after vitrectomy and gas injection, the intraocular pressure can be more safely adjusted by gas removal than by immediate reopening of the filter. Eventual reoperation for intraocular pressure control may be necessary.

The presence of a mobile intraocular lens (especially an anterior chamber lens with iris fixation), which threatens to touch the cornea following choroidal hemorrhage with anterior chamber shallowing, should also prompt surgical drainage and re-formation of the anterior chamber. Pre-placement of stay sutures anterior to an iris-fixated pseudophakos is a prudent precaution in high-risk eyes.

12-7

HYPHEMA

Mild to moderate bleeding into the anterior chamber from the wound or subconjunctival space is usually best left alone. Irrigation may be attempted but seldom completely clears the blood. Hyphema of modest degree during the first few days after filtering surgery usually clears spontaneously. Massive subconjunctival hemorrhage may (rarely) occur, with back-bleeding into the eye during wound closure. Removal of blood from the subconjunctival space and fistula is desirable and may require reopening the conjunctival wound or Tenon's capsule. Recent reports have suggested that thromboplastin activating factor (TPA) may have fruitful application to clearing acute hemorrhages and fibrin from filtering blebs or fistulas.

Minimal bleeding from the region of Schlemm's canal during excision of the scleral block in trabeculectomy procedures often stops spontaneously or after pressure is applied. Persistent or vigorous bleeding that may be from adjacent ciliary body or iris following iridectomy may be cauterized with care to avoid lens injury. The trabeculectomy flap should not be cauterized because it can shrink markedly, making wound closure difficult.

12-8

LATE BLEEDING

Bleeding into the anterior chamber or bleb from exposed small vessels in or around the scleral fistula can occur months to years after surgery. Microhyphema from such bleeding can explain sudden intraocular pressure rise in what has been a well-controlled eye. Application of a large Goldmann or equivalent gonioscopy lens, which compresses episcleral vessels, can be used to transiently increase pressure in the scleral vessels and may demonstrate the bleeding site gonioscopically. Once identified, application of the argon laser to the abnormal vessels may obliterate them and prevent recurrence of hemorrhage.

12-9

PREPLACED PARACENTESIS TRACT

It is desirable to routinely place a paracentesis tract temporally at the edge of the clear cornea, using a beveled incision paralleling the iris. This opening provides access to the anterior chamber for instillation of a viscoelastic substance, air, or balanced salt solution and may be used postoperatively if necessary to re-form or deepen the anterior chamber at the slit lamp.

12-10

CONJUNCTIVAL BUTTONHOLES

Buttonholes can be minimized by use of nontoothed forceps during conjunctival dissection. Careful inspection of the wound at the end of the procedure may reveal obvious defects in wound closure or conjunctival tears away from the primary incision. Seidel testing while injecting balanced salt solution into the anterior chamber through a paracentesis tract to expand the bleb is desirable and is likely to reveal significant wound leaks or unrecognized conjunctival holes. Repair of conjunctival buttonholes or wound leaks can best be accomplished with running or pursestring sutures with small-caliber "vascular" taper-point needles after routine closure of the primary wound.

12-11

SHALLOW OR FLAT ANTERIOR CHAMBER

The anterior chamber is usually of normal depth by 24 hours after trabeculectomy. Slight shallowing of the anterior chamber usually reverses itself over a few days with only routine use of cycloplegics. Marked shallowing with apposition between the peripheral iris and the cornea may be due to overfiltration or excessive leakage through the surgical fistula. Compression over the flap at the slit lamp may reveal immediate deepening of the chamber in such cases. Pressure patching or a tamponade device (Simmons' shell) may accelerate chamber deepening in such cases.

Persistent shallowing for many days, apparently due to overfiltration, may also be reversed by injecting air or a viscoelastic substance into the anterior chamber, temporarily occluding the fistula internally.

Persistent marked shallowing of the anterior chamber associated with hypotony is often accompanied by choroidal effusion. If large choroidal effusions occur and persist 10 to 14 days postoperatively, surgical drainage may be necessary, along with anterior chamber re-formation. Re-formation of the anterior chamber alone in such cases with air, balanced salt solution, or viscoelastic material may not be possible without drainage of the choroidal effusion and usually does not effect a lasting cure. B-scan ultrasound is useful to exclude the presence of hemorrhage in the effusion. Rarely, diffuse choroidal effusion without bullous elevation is demonstrable only by ultrasound and may explain forward displacement of the lens–iris diaphragm. Extreme shallowing of the anterior chamber with threatened or actual lens–cornea touch (or pseudophakos–cornea touch) requires urgent correction, usually surgical, to prevent corneal decompensation.

12-12

WOUND LEAK

Leakage of aqueous directly into the tear film is an obvious explanation for a shallow or flat anterior chamber postoperatively. Direct inspection of the conjunctival wound, whether limbus-based or fornix-based, often reveals a dehiscence or gap in the closure. Seidel testing with direct application of a wet fluorescein strip to the wound is very helpful in identifying leaks. Small leaks around sutures often close without treatment. Leaks with definite streaming of aqueous may be treated with pressure patching for 24 to 48 hours and sometimes seal. Most definite leaks require suturing and should be repaired promptly to ensure maintenance of as large a filtration area as possible. Anterior leaks with fornix-based conjunctival flaps usually require additional sutures in the anterior edges of the scleral flap to ensure leak closure. Tissue glue, advocated by some, may cause intense inflammation and irritation. Cautery with chemicals or heat is more likely to enlarge than shrink a conjunctival wound leak. Small-caliber tapered needles are ideal for postoperative wound-leak repair, which can sometimes be accomplished with topical anesthesia at the slit lamp or with an operating microscope.

12-13

CHRONIC LEAKING BLEB

Rarely, filtration blebs may rupture or leak when thin areas break down months to years after surgery. Otherwise-unexplained irritation in an eye with an established filtration bleb should prompt an examination for a leak. Providing no conjunctival or lid disease predisposes the eye to infection, small leaks may be observed, with or without antibiotic treatment, and many eventually close spontaneously. Surgical repair in some cases necessitates major dissection and mobilization of surrounding conjunctiva and excision of thin, avascular tissue or closure of the previous fistula and reoperation at another site.

12-14

ELEVATED INTRAOCULAR PRESSURE

Elevation of intraocular pressure, even above preoperative levels, may be apparent a few hours after surgery or on the first postoperative day. Usually, the rise in intraocular pressure is due to fibrin or blood occluding the trabeculectomy cleft. Viscoelastic materials may also contribute to transient elevation of intraocular pressure. With a limbus-based wound, gentle massage or distortion of the scleral wound edges through the conjunctiva may effect relief and bleb formation. Caution should be exercised in manipulating a fornix-based wound until 48 to 72 hours postoperatively because it is more easily disrupted. Venting of the anterior chamber via the paracentesis tract by depression of the posterior edge of the wound with a sterile needle at the slit lamp provides temporary (1 to 2 hours) control of intraocular pressure. If the pressure remains unacceptably elevated through the second postoperative day and no bleb is present, consideration may be given to releasing the scleral sutures by laser (laser suture lysis).

Intraocular pressure elevation occurring postoperatively despite a well-formed bleb after beginning topical steroids may be due to steroid response. Discontinuing steroids may effect gradual lowering of intraocular pressure over the next few days. Temporary use of topical antiglaucoma medications (beta blockers, apraclonidine) or carbonic anhydrase inhibitors may be necessary.

12-15

DELLEN

Dellen formation is likely if the conjunctival bleb remains sharply elevated at the limbus for days following surgery or evolves as an elevated encapsulated structure near the corneal margin. Most remain moderate and disappear as the bleb flattens postoperatively. Frequent use of artificial tears or patching is helpful. Permanent stromal scarring is possible if dellen persist, and occasional patients have prolonged discomfort and irritation. Intervention to flatten the bleb is seldom necessary because most dellen respond to conservative management and intervention risks loss of filtration function. Chem-

ical cautery (trichloracetic acid), cauterization of the surface, delimiting external sutures, or reoperation and partial closure of the scleral opening may all be considered if several months of conservative management fail to provide relief.

12-16

MALIGNANT GLAUCOMA

Malignant glaucoma (ciliary block, aqueous misdirection) should be suspected when the anterior chamber is shallow or flat and intraocular pressure elevated. In the vast majority of cases, no obvious choroidal expansion is detected clinically or by ultrasound. A visible anterior bowing of the posterior hyaloid may accompany the forward displacement of the lens–iris diaphragm. The mechanism in this disorder may include impaction of gel vitreous between the equator of the lens and the ciliary processes and accumulation of aqueous behind the posterior hyaloid.

Approximately 50% of these patients respond to vigorous medical treatment with cycloplegics (atropine) and hyperosmotics. Some authorities advocate the frequent application of sympathomimetics (Neo-Synephrine) and systemic use of carbonic anhydrase inhibitors. Those patients responding to medical therapy should be maintained on cycloplegics for several weeks thereafter.

Some aphakic or pseudophakic eyes that do not respond promptly (24 to 48 hours) to medical therapy and have clear media may respond to disruption of the posterior or anterior hyaloid with an Nd:YAG laser. Disruption of the vitreous face and posterior hyaloid and vitreous tap using a needle inserted through the pars plana always effects at least temporary relief and sometimes is curative. Complete pars plana vitrectomy in aphakic or pseudophakic eyes may be the most definitive method of cure. Partial (core) vitrectomy may be effective without lens injury in phakic eyes. Complete pars plana vitrectomy and lensectomy may be necessary if the site of block is near the equator of the lens. Intracapsular lens extraction with planned vitrectomy has been advocated in the past. The common denominator of definitive treatment of malignant glaucoma is removal of sufficient vitreous to restore free flow of aqueous into the anterior chamber.

Pupillary block due to posterior synechiae or fibrin, blood, or vitreous occlusion of the peripheral iridectomy could also explain forward displacement of the iris (bombé) occurring postoperatively.

12-17

INFLAMMATION

Rarely, delayed inflammation (uveitis and choroidal effusion) may follow otherwise-successful filtering surgery and may include shallowing of the anterior chamber. Treatment with cycloplegics and topical and systemic steroids may be indicated.

12-18

INFECTION

Early or delayed endophthalmitis after filtering surgery is surprisingly rare, perhaps due to the usual external direction of aqueous flow. Late postoperative endophthalmitis may follow traumatic bleb rupture, with infection of the bleb externally followed by intraocular spread of the process. Early, vigorous antibiotic therapy with both topical and systemic medication may arrest the infection and avoid endophthalmitis. Hospital admission and close monitoring of patients suspected of having infected filtering blebs are mandatory to ensure prompt control of the infection. Smears and cultures from the involved area should be obtained immediately before starting broad-spectrum topical and systemic antibiotics. Smear and culture results can be used to modify the antibiotic therapy thereafter. Vitreous and anterior chamber tap and intraocular antibiotics should be employed if progression of the infection into intraocular spaces is suspected.

Infection of a bleb, even when promptly sterilized with appropriate antibiotic therapy, almost invariably destroys the bleb's function. Filtering surgery at another site may be necessary once the patient recovers from the infection. Preliminary followup has suggested that the risk of late endophthalmitis after filtering surgery is increased in patients who receive 5-fluorouracil postoperatively.

12-19

CLINICAL PEARLS

Attention to several clinical pearls may enhance the rate of success and diminish the rate of complications:

1. Assess the risk of choroidal hemorrhage prior to surgery and plan for its management in high-risk patients. Consider pre-placement of a scleral fistula in both lower quadrants before opening the eye, and leave the fistulas open in case choroidal hemorrhage occurs postoperatively.

2. Use a Flieringa ring or other support device to minimize scleral distortion intraoperatively in high-risk patients and when anterior vitrectomy may be likely.

3. Avoid sudden drops in intraocular pressure. The pressure may be lowered by preoperative hyperosmotics or retrobulbar anesthesia and further gradually lowered via a paracentesis tract. Consider an infusion line to help control intraocular pressure during surgery. Place a paracentesis tract for intraoperative or postoperative use.

4. Leave the eye at normal or slightly elevated intraocular pressure at the conclusion of surgery. Viscoelastic materials or air may help prevent profound hypotony for several hours after surgery. High pressure is likely during the first several hours after surgery if the scleral flap is tightly sutured.

5. Otherwise-unexplained pain in the operated eye during the first few days after surgery should prompt a search for choroidal bleeding, including ultrasound if necessary.

6. Shallowing of the anterior chamber and hypotony postoperatively should prompt a careful search for wound leak and choroidal expansion.

12-20

SUMMARY

The most serious intraoperative complications of glaucoma filtering surgery include choroidal hemorrhage and buttonholes of the conjunctiva. The risk of intraoperative choroidal hemorrhage can be decreased by avoiding distortion of the globe and minimizing the period of profound hypotony. Serious postoperative complications of filtering surgery include delayed choroidal hemorrhage, malignant glaucoma, flat chamber, late wound leak, and infection. The risk of any of these will be decreased by meticulous intraoperative surgical technique and conscientious postoperative care. Hypotony during the first few hours after trabeculectomy can be minimized by adjusting the scleral flap sutures to allow minimal aqueous leak or by using a tight scleral closure and planned laser suture lysis or adjustable (removable) sutures postoperatively. Vigorous cycloplegia and topical steroids are important.

BIBLIOGRAPHY

Agarwal SP, Hendeles S: Risk of sudden visual loss following trabeculectomy in advanced primary open-angle glaucoma. *Br J Ophthalmol* 1986;**70**:97–99.

Blondeau P, Phelps CD: Trabeculectomy vs thermo-sclerostomy: a randomized prospective clinical trial. *Arch Ophthalmol* 1981;**99**:810–816.

Cantor LB, Katz LJ, Spaeth GL: Complications of surgery in glaucoma: suprachoroidal expulsive hemorrhage in patients undergoing intraocular surgery. *Ophthalmology* 1985;**92**: 1266–1270.

Frenkel REP, Shin DH: Prevention and management of delayed suprachoroidal hemorrhage after filtration surgery. *Arch Ophthalmol* 1986; **104**:1459–1463.

Givens K, Shields MB: Suprachoroidal hemorrhage after glaucoma filtering surgery. *Am J Ophthalmol* 1987;**103**:689–694.

Hoskins HD Jr, Kass MA: *Becker-Shaffer's Diagnosis and Therapy of the Glaucomas.* St Louis: CV Mosby Co; 1989:572–582.

Katz LJ, Spaeth GL: Filtration surgery. In: Ritch R, Shields MB, Krupin T, eds: *The Glaucomas.* St Louis: CV Mosby Co; 1989:653–696.

Kolker AE: Discussion of steroid-induced ocular hypertension in patients with filtering blebs. *Ophthalmology* 1980;**87**:243–244.

Kolker AE: Visual prognosis in advanced glaucoma: a comparison of medical and surgical therapy for retention of vision in 101 eyes with advanced glaucoma. *Trans Am Ophthalmol Soc* 1977;**75**:539–555.

Minckler DS, Shammas A, Wilcox M, et al: Experimental studies of aqueous filtration using the Molteno implant. *Trans Am Ophthalmol Soc* 1987;**85**:368–392.

Commentary

Richard A. Lewis, MD

Dr Minckler has provided a comprehensive summary of complications during and after filtration surgery. Another complication occurs approximately 4 to 8 weeks postoperatively. A large, dome-shaped, encapsulated bleb is often associated with marked elevation of intraocular pressure and what appears to be a very well-functioning filter. The so-called encapsulated bleb is usually a self-limited condition. Because the complication is associated with marked intraocular pressure elevation, aqueous suppressants are necessary to reduce intraocular pressure. Most often the medications are necessary for only a brief period of time, approximately 2 to 4 weeks. Although the etiology of the encapsulated bleb is unclear, it appears to come at a time of bleb remodeling, accompanied by full aqueous production. It has been estimated that more than 90% of the time the condition is self-limited. Occasionally, the bleb will need to be surgically remodeled, with excision of the encapsulated tissue. The use of 5-fluorouracil in this setting is recommended, although its efficacy is not proven.

CHAPTER 13

Assessment and Management of Filtering Blebs

E. Michael Van Buskirk, MD

The goal of glaucoma filtration surgery is to create a permanent fistula from the anterior chamber to the subconjunctival space. This fistula effectively bypasses the obstructed glaucomatous conventional aqueous humor outflow pathways and diverts the aqueous humor into a subconjunctival reservoir, the filtration bleb. Filtration blebs take on a wide variety of clinical characteristics depending on the type of filtration procedure, the surgical technique, the underlying ocular disease state, and the inherent endogenous wound-healing characteristics of the individual patient.

13-1

BLEB CHARACTERISTICS

The bleb's clinical appearance does not always reflect its function, but some clinical signs are associated with good function and others are associated with poor function. In general, blebs that are working well tend to be diffuse, covering at least a quadrant of the global surface. They tend to be low, not markedly distended. They often have a watery, succulent, translucent appearance and are relatively avascular (Figure 13-1). The most useful clinical sign of good bleb function is the development of fine, confluent microcysts within the conjunctival epithelium. Conversely, when a bleb is localized to a small area of the global surface, the conjunctiva is usually bound down to the underlying episclera by fibrotic tissue, confining aqueous absorption to a small area. This can be associated with marked distention of the conjunctiva and subconjunctival tissues in that area because the bleb area is under

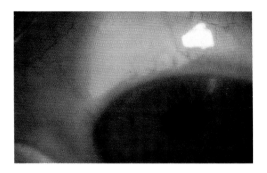

Figure 13-1 *A well-functioning bleb: low, diffuse, succulent, translucent, and relatively avascular.*

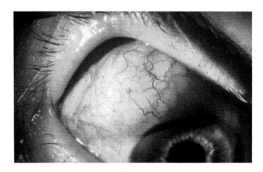

Figure 13-2 *A poorly functioning bleb: localized, distended, thick, and hypervascular.*

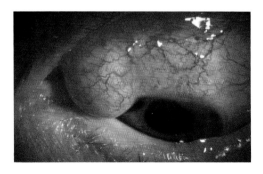

Figure 13-3 *An encapsulated filtration bleb.*

increased intraocular pressure (Figure 13-2). Such blebs tend to be hypervascular and to function poorly. On the other hand, a bleb that is paper-thin and transparent rather than translucent is associated with low intraocular pressure but tends to leak and is susceptible to infection. A bleb that is completely collapsed and flat indicates an obstructed filtration fistula and poor filtration.

13-2

CAUSES OF POOR FILTRATION

Although the vast majority of filtration procedures performed in uncomplicated open-angle glaucoma result in a well-functioning filtration bleb with low intraocular pressure, endogenous factors in some patients lead to an increased incidence of failure. Often, these factors are not specifically identifiable but are related to the wound-healing properties of the individual patient.

Filtration surgery fails more often in black patients than in white patients. The aged patient shows less tendency toward impermeable scar formation than the young patient. Children under the age of 10 carry an especially poor prognosis. Patients with secondary glaucoma tend to do more poorly than patients with primary glaucoma, particularly patients who have uveitis or ocular neovascularization or who have undergone previous intraocular surgery. Patients who are aphakic and have had vitrectomy or retinal detachment surgery or who have had extensive conjunctival scarring tend to carry a particularly poor prognosis.

In addition, some iatrogenic surgical or technical factors lead to increased fibrosis and failure. These include rough surgical technique, excess cautery, excess bleeding, or excessive intraocular manipulation. Two common technical errors leading to failure of limbus-based trabeculectomy are making the conjunctival incision too far anterior, thereby localizing the bleb to a small perilimbal area, and making the transscleral incision too far posterior, entering over the ciliary body. Further, suturing the scleral flap so tightly that no fistula ever develops is perhaps the most common and most neglected cause of the failed filter.

Poorly functioning filtration blebs can be divided into two general categories: failure within the bleb itself and obstruction of the transscleral fistula. Thus, the patient with a failing filter should be examined thoroughly to classify anatomically the pathogenesis of filtration failure.

13-3

FAILURE OF THE BLEB

13-3-1 Encapsulated Bleb

Encapsulation of the filtration bleb is the most common cause of failure during the first 6-week postoperative period. The encapsulated bleb clinically appears as an elevated, dome-like structure extending several millimeters in height above the global surface, with a sharply defined, often vascular border binding the subconjunctival tissues to the episclera (Figure 13-3). The conjunctiva is markedly distended, tightly stretched over the dome of a subconjunctival impermeable fibrotic wall. The encapsulated bleb appears quite vascular during the first few weeks, becoming thinner and less vascular with the passage of time.

13-3-1-1 Medical Management The vast majority of encapsulated blebs eventually function spontaneously without surgical intervention, but many weeks may be required. In the meantime, patience and perseverance are required on the part of both surgeon and patient, as well as continuing vigilance for preservation of the optic nerve. Topical anti-inflammatory drugs such as corticosteroids likely inhibit further fibrosis, but are not dramatic in their effect. Aqueous suppressant agents such as topical beta blockers are sometimes effective in reducing the intraocular pressure.

Digital compression seems to be effective in some patients. Massage can be performed directly over the bleb when encapsulation occurs, especially if a trabeculectomy has been performed. The conjunctiva is anesthetized with topical proparacaine. A moistened cotton stick should be directly applied to the dome of the encapsulated area, with the patient looking downward (Figure 13-4). The bleb should be compressed for 10 to 20 seconds. During compression, the trabeculectomy flap, forced into the scleral bed, serves as a flap valve, preventing the retrogression of aqueous into the anterior

Figure 13-4 *Direct cotton stick massage/compression of an encapsulated bleb, compressing the trabeculectomy flap into its bed and forcing trapped aqueous into the subconjunctival space.*

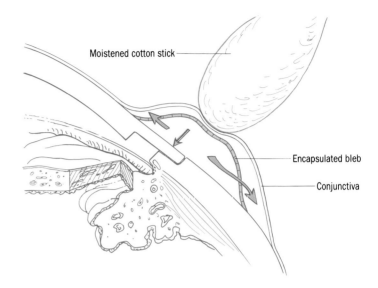

Moistened cotton stick

Encapsulated bleb

Conjunctiva

chamber. This will force the entrapped aqueous through the encapsulated wall into the surrounding subconjunctival space. The subconjunctival expression of fluid through the encapsulated wall can be identified adjacent to the encapsulated zone at the slit lamp during the compression process. The eye may then be compressed along the limbus inferiorly to reinflate the encapsulated area and reduce the intraocular pressure. This process should be repeated by the surgeon at the slit lamp 2 to 3 times weekly until spontaneous filtration occurs.

13-3-1-2 Surgical Revision   Surgical revision should be delayed as long as possible because the vast majority of encapsulated blebs will function spontaneously without

revision. The surgeon must also bear in mind that any revision can simply recycle the process, with the bleb again becoming encapsulated a few weeks after the revision. However, in some cases, the eye is unable to withstand the elevated intraocular pressure for a sustained period of time because of advanced optic disc changes.

Two surgical techniques are effective: incisional revision (or needling) and excisional revision. Needling is easier to perform but successfully restores filtration only about 50% of the time. A limbal intracameral paracentesis should be performed. Balanced salt solution should be injected into the subconjunctival space with a 23-gauge needle inserted at the periphery of the bleb. This elevates the conjunctiva away from the encapsulated wall (Figure 13-5A). At the operating microscope, the surgeon will then be able to identify the firm, grayish fibrotic wall of the encapsulated area in the subconjunctival space. A Ziegler-type needle knife may then be inserted into the needle puncture in the subconjunctival space or passed under conjunctiva to engage the encapsulated area (Figure 13-5B). The knife should be passed through the encapsulated area, exiting on the opposite side, and then gradually directed posteriorly to create an internal incision of about 4 to 5 clock hours along the posterior edge of the base of the encapsulated area. The knife is then withdrawn. The incision should be closed with a single horizontal mattress suture with 10-0 nylon. Aqueous will gush forth from within the cavity of the encapsulation into subconjunctival space. The eye will become very soft. The anterior chamber can then be deepened to slightly greater than normal depth through the paracentesis tract and the eye treated postoperatively with cycloplegics, topical steroids, and antibiotics. Massage should be instituted as soon as the spontaneous intraocular pressure exceeds 15 mm Hg or if there is any sign that encapsulation has recurred.

An alternative approach is to reopen the original conjunctival incision only to the level of Tenon's capsule. The conjunctival flap should then be carefully dissected anteriorly toward the encapsulated fibrotic wall. The conjunctiva should be gently dissected over the dome of the encapsulated wall to the limbus, and the encapsulated wall completely excised using Vannas scissors (Figure 13-6). The flap should then be repositioned to its normal anatomic position, and the wound closed in the conventional manner. As with nee-

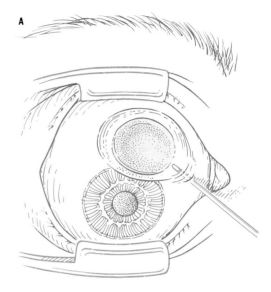

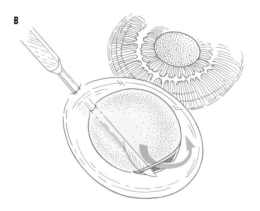

Figure 13-5 *Surgical revision of an encapsulated bleb. (A) Incisional revision (needling). (B) Internal incision with a Ziegler-type knife.*

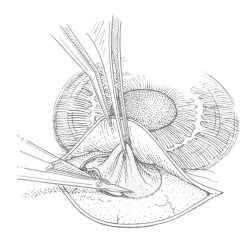

Figure 13-6 *Excisional revision of an encapsulated bleb.*

dling, the eye will become very soft as soon as the encapsulated area is opened and the anterior chamber should be deepened through the previously placed paracentesis tract, as described above.

13-3-2 Leaking Bleb

Blebs may leak from the bleb cavity to the conjunctival surface under three circumstances:

1. A buttonhole or tear of the conjunctiva during surgery.

2. Inadequate wound closure at the time of surgery with postoperative wound leak.

3. Late leakage of a thin-walled cystic bleb.

Conjunctival buttonholes can be closed at the time of surgery or postoperatively using a 10-0 nylon horizontal mattress suture to achieve a fluid-tight closure (Figure 13-7). Small wound leaks sometimes close spontaneously, but if the bleb has collapsed and a gap in the wound is visible, the gap is best closed with a 10-0 nylon mattress suture. Most important for closing conjunctival wound leaks is the use of an atraumatic, tapered, noncutting microvascular needle with 10-0 nylon or polypropylene (Ethicon BV 4-100). This type of needle prevents the creation of further conjunctival holes with passage of the needle.

Most commonly, a leaking bleb occurs late in the postoperative period, sometimes many years after the surgery, and is associated with a paper-thin, transparent cystic bleb wall. In some cases, the only manifestation is a positive Seidel test. Despite a positive Seidel test, an eye that is

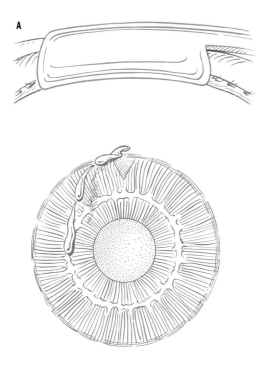

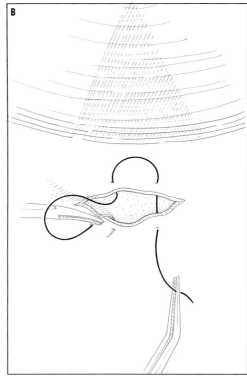

Figure 13-7 *(A) A leaking filtration bleb from a limbal buttonhole. (B) Horizontal mattress closure of a limbal buttonhole with a tapered needle. (C) Completed horizontal mattress closure.*

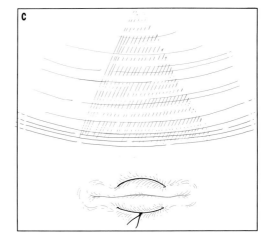

not hypotonous and that has an anterior chamber of normal depth needs no special treatment except for more intensive and regular followup. In other cases, topical or systemic aqueous suppressants such as beta blockers or carbonic anhydrase inhibitors reduce aqueous flow sufficiently to allow the leak to close spontaneously. Long-term topical antibiotic therapy can be considered.

If a visible perforation is evident or if hypotony (shallow anterior chamber, variable visual acuity, choroidal detachment, macular edema, or disc edema) occurs, surgical revision is indicated. Because of the thin, diaphanous nature of the conjunctival wall in cystic limbal blebs, these blebs rarely can be repaired with a simple pursestring suture. A more definitive approach is to excise the entire cystic area. The surrounding conjunctiva should then be undermined posteriorly (Figure 13-8). A small, very shallow keratectomy groove approximately the width of the cystic area should be prepared at the corneal limbus. The newly created conjunctival flap should then be advanced anteriorly and sutured into the keratectomy groove with interrupted horizontal mattress sutures. If the conjunctival flap is too small or too tight, a relaxing incision may be made posteriorly in the region of the original conjunctival incision. The flap may then be advanced to the limbus. Finally, the posterior lip of the relaxing incision should be undermined sufficiently to close the posterior wound. Such blebs should be monitored very carefully postoperatively for reduction of bleb function.

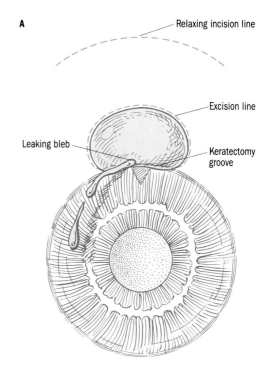

A

Relaxing incision line

Excision line

Leaking bleb

Keratectomy groove

Figure 13-8 *(A) A perforated, transparent cystic bleb. (B) Excision of a cystic leaking filtration bleb at the limbus. (C) Undermining the conjunctiva between the site of the excised leaking area and the superior/posterior relaxing incision. (D) Shallow keratectomy groove at the limbal periphery to receive the anterior edge of conjunctiva. (E) Closure of the limbus to the keratectomy groove with interrupted horizontal mattress sutures and closure of the superior/posterior relaxing incision.*

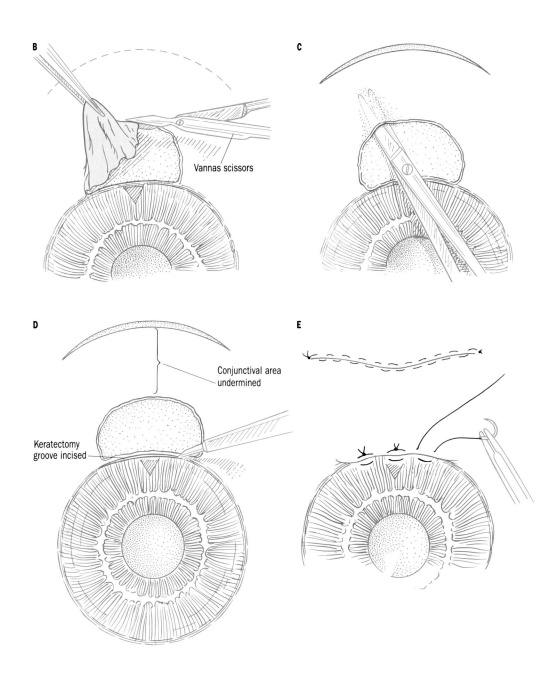

B

Vannas scissors

C

D

Conjunctival area
undermined

Keratectomy
groove incised

E

OBSTRUCTION OF THE FISTULA

Filtration fistulas can be obstructed at four sites (Figure 13-9):

1. Starting externally, an episcleral cap-like membrane can overgrow the external opening whether a full-thickness or partial-thickness scleral flap procedure was performed. (These episcleral membranes bridge the gap between fistula obstruction and bleb failure, but are discussed here, under fistular occlusion, for convenience.)

2. The scleral flap can be sutured so tightly to the scleral bed or can gradually become so scarred in the scleral bed that it obstructs the fistula at that level.

3. In rare cases, progressive ingrowth of the fibroblasts can fill in the transscleral portion of the fistula.

4. The internal opening of the fistula on the anterior chamber side can be obstructed with a variety of thin-walled membranes deriving from the surrounding corneal scleral tissue or from the iris, ciliary body, lens, or even vitreous humor.

13-4-1 Gray Bleb

Proliferation of episcleral membranes blocking the external opening of the fistula is a common cause of the failed filter (Figure 13-9A). These membranes create a readily identifiable clinical picture in which a very small, slightly elevated, firm bleb is localized to a few millimeters around the fistular site. No microcystic changes occur within the conjunctiva because the aqueous humor is entrapped behind the membrane. The conjunctiva is usually mobile and can be slid over a grayish, glistening fibrotic membrane readily seen in the subconjunctival space. The episcleral membrane bleb rarely responds to digital compression or to topical medical therapy, but these modalities are best tried first.

In the absence of a therapeutic response, the gray bleb/episcleral cap requires surgical revision. In some cases, the bleb is sufficiently identifiable to be incised by the needling approach discussed earlier. Most, in my experience, require an excisional approach. The original conjunctival incision is opened and the conjunctiva is carefully dissected anteriorly to be reflected over the cornea as with conventional filtration surgery. At the filtration site, a paper-thin, firm, and impermeable membrane can be identified overlying the external opening (Figure 13-10). A paracentesis should be performed before this membrane is penetrated. The membrane should then be excised with fine scissors such as the Vannas (see Figure 13-7). Immediately, aqueous will gush forth from the fistula and the eye will become very soft. The conjunctival flap should be re-placed to its normal anatomic position, and the conjunctival incision closed. The anterior chamber should then be deepened to slightly greater than normal depth through the paracentesis tract. Because

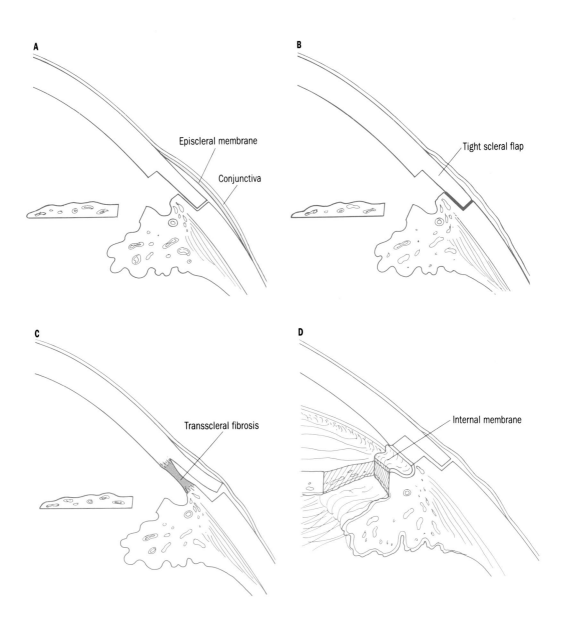

Figure 13-9 *The four sites of obstructed filtration fistulas. (A) Episcleral membrane. (B) Tight scleral flap. (C) Transscleral fibrosis. (D) Internal fistular membrane.*

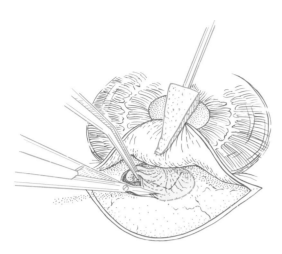

Figure 13-10 *Episcleral membrane covering the external opening of a filtration fistula.*

these episcleral membranes result from excess fibroblast proliferation, the surgeon may want to consider subconjunctival 5-fluorouracil therapy or other vigorous antimetabolite therapy to prevent their recurrence.

13-4-2 Tight Scleral Flap

Perhaps the most commonly unrecognized cause of the failed filter after partial-thickness (trabeculectomy) procedures is the tight scleral flap (see Figure 13-9B). The tight scleral flap may occur either early in the postoperative period or late.

In the early postoperative period, the flap either may become adherent to the underlying scleral bed because of fibrin or other blood products or may be sutured so tightly that no filtration can occur. In either circumstance, no bleb is evident. In the first instance, the flap may be loosened by gentle manipulation with one or two cotton sticks overlying the flap and the adjacent scleral tissue. In the second, one or more sutures should be lysed. Lysis can be easily accomplished with an argon laser. A Hoskins-type contact lens or the triangular facet of a Zeiss gonioscopy lens should be gently but firmly applied to the conjunctiva overlying the scleral flap, gently squeezing all blood and tissue fluid from the conjunctiva. As a result, the 10-0 nylon suture will stand out brightly against the surrounding white sclera (Figure 13-11). The suture can then be readily incised by a 50-micron beam at about 500 mW for 0.1 second. Exposure can be titrated to sever the suture.

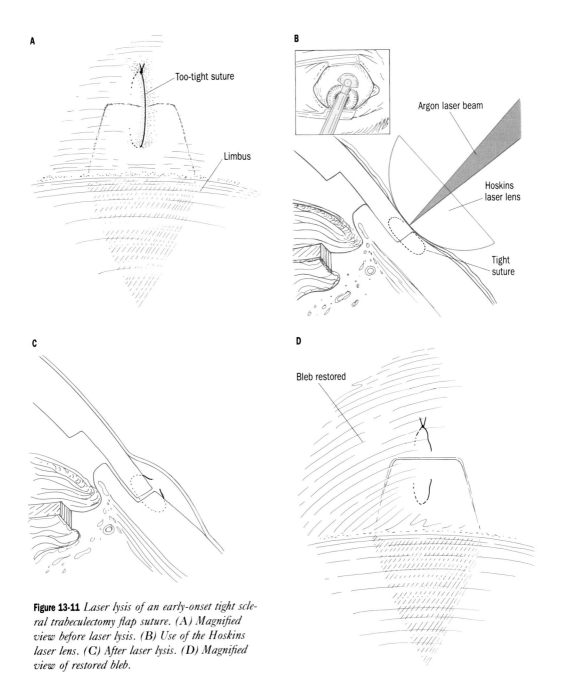

Figure 13-11 *Laser lysis of an early-onset tight scleral trabeculectomy flap suture. (A) Magnified view before laser lysis. (B) Use of the Hoskins laser lens. (C) After laser lysis. (D) Magnified view of restored bleb.*

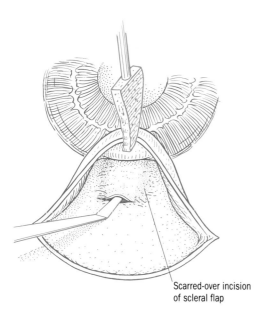

Scarred-over incision
of scleral flap

Figure 13-12 *Surgical reopening for a late-onset tight scleral flap obstructing the filtration fistula.*

The tight scleral flap can also occur in the late postoperative period (months or years) as a process of gradual fibrosis, the flap gradually settling down into the scleral bed and becoming adherent to it. This situation is usually associated with a flat, virtually nonexistent filtration bleb of long-standing failure. It can also be identified gonioscopically. The sharp edges of the internal opening of the filtration fistula are readily visible, but the fistula is covered by the white scleral flap adherent along its posterior edge. The scleral flap can be loosened from the underlying scleral bed by applying Nd:YAG laser energy at the cleavage plane between the flap and the scleral bed along the posterior edge of the fistula, but this procedure is rarely successful. In other cases, the conjunctival incision needs to be reopened, the conjunctival flap dissected anteriorly, and the scleral flap raised in a manner similar to the original trabeculectomy (Figure 13-12).

13-4-3 Transscleral Fibrosis

In very rare cases, the borders of the internal aspect of the transscleral fistula between the anterior chamber and the scleral flap becomes gradually blurred or rounded, as viewed with gonioscopy (see Figure 3-9C). This occurs because of an ingrowth of fibroblasts from the surrounding tissue, with the gradual filling in of the fistula. At first, only the margins of the fistula are blurred, but ultimately the entire fistula becomes filled, giving it a dimple-like appearance (Figure 13-13). At this stage, the fistula can sometimes be reopened by multiple applications of the

A

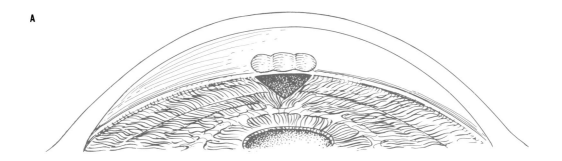

B

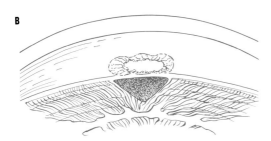

Figure 13-13 *Transscleral fibrosis (diminishing-dimple syndrome). (A–D) The progressive obstruction of the filtration fistula.*

C

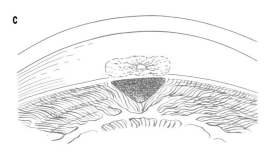

D

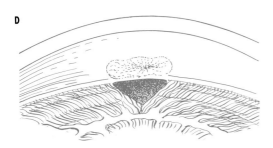

A

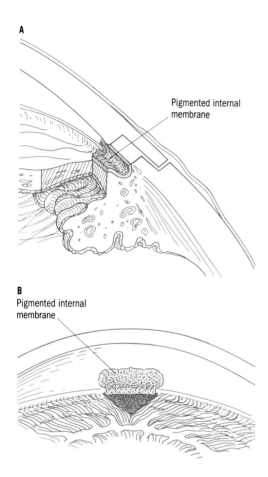

Pigmented internal
membrane

B
Pigmented internal
membrane

Figure 13-14 *Membranous occlusion of the internal fistular opening. (A) Lateral view. (B) Gonioscopic view.*

Nd:YAG laser. If neglected, the fistula will be completely filled in by fibrosis and gonioscopically no fistula will be evident at all.

13-4-4 Internal Fistular Membrane

Membranes from surrounding intraocular structures can overgrow the internal fistular opening (see Figure 13-9D). These membranes can derive from the surrounding cornea and sclera, leaving a waxed-paper–like membrane over the fistula, and can be relatively easily reopened with the Nd:YAG laser. Iris epithelium or ciliary body epithelium can also proliferate to overgrow the internal opening (Figure 13-14). These membranes can be reopened with either the argon or the Nd:YAG laser. Lens components, especially in patients who have had extracapsular cataract surgery, may also overgrow the internal opening. These are usually flaps of capsule that simply come to lie over the internal opening as a flap valve, but in other cases these can serve as scaffolding for the proliferation of tissues into the fistula. These also sometimes respond to Nd:YAG laser reopening. Finally, in the aphakic patient, vitreous can migrate through the peripheral iridectomy to occlude the fistula. These relatively broad bands of vitreous cannot be readily removed with the Nd:YAG laser. Moreover, the Nd:YAG laser may cause undue traction on the vitreous and lead to peripheral retinal tears. For this reason, I recommend anterior vitrectomy to remove the vitreous from the anterior chamber and from the fistula. When performed early, blebs can be readily restored.

13-5

SUMMARY

Anatomic identification of bleb failure pathogenesis helps in guiding management. Failing blebs may occur because of fibrosis within the bleb itself or because of blockage of flow through the transscleral fistula. Many failed blebs eventually function spontaneously or can be restored with appropriate medical or surgical therapy. The surgeon should avoid the temptation to give up on a potentially salvageable bleb and should preserve the remaining conjunctiva in case further surgery becomes necessary.

BIBLIOGRAPHY

Skuta GL, Parrish RK II: Wound healing in glaucoma filtering surgery. *Surv Ophthalmol* 1987;**32**:149–170.

Van Buskirk EM: Occluded filtration fistulas: diagnosis and laser treatment. *Trans First Scientific Meeting of Am Glaucoma Soc* 1988; chap 21.

Commentary

Richard P. Mills, MD

Surgically created filtration blebs go through a maturation process as the three phases of wound healing progress. In the earliest phase following trabeculectomy, aqueous flow into the subconjunctival space is restricted only by the resistance of the sutured superficial scleral flap, so the anterior chamber may shallow or (rarely) flatten. Within a few days, however, the conjunctival and subconjunctival tissues become stiffer, as can be demonstrated if the surgeon attempts to irrigate fluid through the paracentesis tract. Generally, the bleb will elevate, but not nearly as dramatically as it did at the conclusion of the operation. During this period, wound leaks—which allow transconjunctival egress of fluid without elevating the bleb—can allow the tissue to stiffen and scar in the collapsed bleb so even when the leak has sealed, an elevated bleb does not form.

If the intraocular pressure normalizes and the anterior chamber remains deep within the first few postoperative days, the superficial scleral flap may be restricting flow and should be loosened mechanically or with laser suture lysis. This maneuver is rarely successful after 7 days and almost never after 10 days, so early recognition is important.

Many blebs develop thickened walls 2 to 10 weeks postoperatively, the extreme examples of which are called *Tenon's cysts*. Given time and the chance to remodel the collagen, most blebs become more permeable to aqueous humor and pressure control is re-established.

Dr Van Buskirk mentions the clusters of fine, translucent, conjunctival epithelial microcysts that are a reliable indicator of bleb function in the late postoperative period. Microcysts should be carefully searched for in the general vicinity of the surgical site, under high magnification with a medium slit width, looking in the retroillumination just adjacent to the slit beam.

Commentary

Donald S. Minckler, MD

This chapter provides a thorough review of the various factors involved in the development of a desirable filtration bleb following glaucoma surgery. The problem of the encapsulated bleb is presented as the major and most frustrating aspect of postoperative management.

A conservative approach to managing these problems is highly recommended because many of them improve with time. Dr Van Buskirk makes excellent points about the process of surgical bleb revision, including the routine placement of a paracentesis tract and the stabilization of the anterior chamber before manipulation of the encapsulated bleb.

The posttrabeculectomy revision (excision of an encapsulated bleb) with the use of 5-fluorouracil is particularly intriguing as a method of dealing with this problem. Only time will tell whether or not this additional manipulation will be useful.

Laser suture lysis is an effective method of modifying the postoperative course of a filtering bleb, either following the initial surgery or during revision if the sutures in the scleral flap are clearly identifiable. Unfortunately, because many patients develop opacity of the conjunctiva or hemorrhage, it is difficult to adequately visualize the sutures in order to break them with the argon laser.

My experience with Nd:YAG laser surgery of partly closed fistulas internally has been extremely disappointing. The rare instances of remarkable, temporary improvement have occurred when a membrane was clearly visible over the internal fistula.

PART IV

Laser and Cyclodestructive Surgery

CHAPTER 14

Argon Laser Trabeculoplasty

Donald S. Minckler, MD

Argon laser trabeculoplasty (ALT) has become an important adjunct to the treatment of open-angle glaucoma. The indications and technique have become relatively standardized since its introduction by Wise and Witter (1979). Complications occurring during or immediately after the procedure have been well characterized (Hoskins et al 1983). The long-term clinical results remain under study, as do the mechanisms by which ALT effects improvement in intraocular pressure control (Schwartz et al 1985, Goldstick and Weinreb 1989).

14-1

INDICATIONS

This procedure is appropriately applied to patients with open-angle glaucoma who cannot be controlled by medical therapy. ALT is under study as primary therapy in an ongoing randomized, prospective trial sponsored by the National Eye Institute (GLT Research Group 1990).

ALT has been extremely useful as an alternative to filtration surgery or as a method of delaying filtration surgery, especially for the systemically fragile elderly patient. The procedure has been relatively successful in primary open-angle glaucoma in patients over 50 years of age and in open-angle glaucoma associated with pseudoexfoliation and pigmentary dispersion (Goldstick and Weinreb 1989).

ALT has had poor success in patients with congenital or juvenile-onset glaucoma, inflammatory glaucoma, and posttraumatic glaucoma with angle-recession injury. The effects are relatively unpredictable in aphakia, pseudophakia, or after multiple previous surgeries. Some studies have found the procedure to have less enduring success in blacks than in whites (Schwartz et al 1985).

14-2

EXPECTATIONS

ALT produces an average decrease in intraocular pressure of 7 to 10 mm Hg (Goldstick and Weinreb 1989). The amount of drop obtained increases as the baseline intraocular pressure increases. The pressure tends to drift back toward the baseline following ALT. The average benefit in intraocular pressure control lasts 3 to 5 years (Schwartz et al 1985). By 5 years after ALT, about 46% of treated patients remain better controlled. The failure rate is approximately 10% per year. Only approximately 30% of patients will be controlled after ALT on reduced topical or systemic medications. Visual field studies have suggested that approximately 26% of patients continue to have field loss despite better control of intraocular pressure after laser treatment (Schultz et al 1987).

14-3

SURGICAL TECHNIQUE

To blunt the rise in intraocular pressure after surgery, preoperative use of pilocarpine, carbonic anhydrase inhibitors, or hyperosmotics has been recommended in patients with extremely advanced optic nerve injury. An alpha adrenergic agonist (apraclonidine) has been approved for topical application before and after laser surgery based on its demonstrated efficacy in preventing spikes of intraocular pressure after laser trabeculoplasty (Robin et al 1987).

Prior to commencing ALT, the surgeon must ensure that the optics of the slit lamp have been adjusted to make his view parfocal with the laser. This can be most easily accomplished by individually adjusting each eyepiece (after first fogging with extra plus) so as to sharply focus the aiming beam on a model target. Observers should wear appropriate eye protectors or remain at least 1.5 m from the target mirror to minimize the risk of accidental retinal burns. The surgeon should not arm the laser or place his foot on the firing pedal until he has established a clear view of the target and aiming beam through the gonioscopic lens to avoid accidental retinal or iris burns in the patient's eye.

Only topical anesthesia with proparacaine (0.5%) is necessary. One eye or both eyes may be treated at the same session. A high-quality gonioscopic lens coated for laser use is mandatory to ensure consistent energy applications. Bubble-free coupling material must be used. The patient should be comfortable and stable. The procedure is usually painless, but the patient may experience vasovagal attacks, including nausea and vomiting. The cornea must be sufficiently clear and free of endothelial pigment to deliver laser energy without obscuring the angle view or producing endothelial or stromal burns.

The surgeon can minimize induced astigmatism in the aiming and treatment

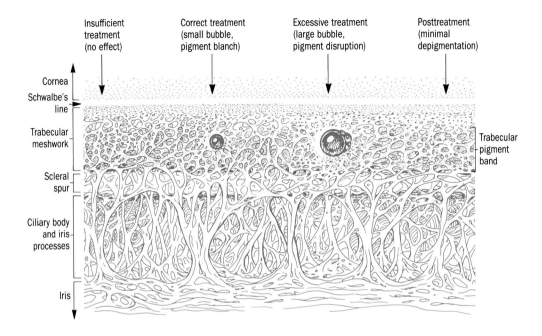

Insufficient treatment (no effect)

Correct treatment (small bubble, pigment blanch)

Excessive treatment (large bubble, pigment disruption)

Posttreatment (minimal depigmentation)

Cornea

Schwalbe's line

Trabecular meshwork

Scleral spur

Ciliary body and iris processes

Iris

Trabecular pigment band

Figure 14-1 *Treatment responses in the trabecular meshwork to light, optimal, and excessive argon laser applications.*

beams by proper positioning of the lens to avoid distortion of the cornea. The laser aiming beam should be sharply focused and round on the target meshwork before application of burns. The gonioscopic view should provide clear access to the target tissue without risk of hitting the iris, and may be improved by asking the patient to look toward the mirror in use.

The principal landmark for orientation in the angle is the scleral spur, which is the only reliable and consistent structure from eye to eye. The pigment band in the posterior meshwork, if present, is a good landmark but can be easily confused by the inexperienced surgeon with pigment along Schwalbe's line. Because the angle is usually wider inferiorly, the surgeon may wish to rotate the mirror to view the angle inferiorly to ensure proper anatomic orientation. Once identified, the scleral spur can be observed around the angle for orientation in other quadrants.

The technique for ALT originally recommended by Wise and Witter (1979) included 100 burns of 50-micron size spaced evenly around the circumference of the trabecular meshwork. Power settings were adjusted to cause minimally detectable pigment blanching or bubble formation (averaging about 800 mW with blue-green argon). The duration of burns recommended remains 0.1 second. Spacing of the burns should allow approximately 25 lesions per quadrant (about 3° between burns).

The ideal target tissue is still thought to be the midmeshwork, most easily identified in patients with some pigment in the trabecular meshwork by straddling the junction between pigmented and nonpigmented meshwork. Many have subsequently modified the technique to treat only 180° of the meshwork initially, electing to defer subsequent treatment of the opposite 180° depending on intraocular pressure response to the first therapy. If no response is noted during the subsequent 4 to 6 weeks, the opposite 180° may be treated (Figures 14-1 and 14-2).

In patients with minimal or no meshwork pigment and no detectable tissue reaction to laser energy in the usual range of power settings, many surgeons will simply select a power (800 to 1200 mW) and proceed with treatment. In patients with variable pigmentation of the meshwork, the power can be continually adjusted during treatment to provide the minimally detectable injury desired.

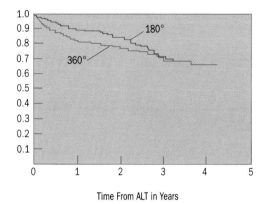

Time From ALT in Years

Figure 14-2 *Graph indicating the cumulative success of argon laser trabeculoplasty comparing 360° treatment to 180° treatment. In this study, patients who had 180° treatment had the opposite 180° treated if intraocular pressure rose to pretreatment levels. Approximately 50% of the initial 180° group had subsequent additional treatment of the remaining 180° of the angle.*
Reprinted by permission from unpublished data by
H. Dunbar Hoskins, Jr, MD, and John Hetherington, MD.

POSTOPERATIVE CARE

Intraocular pressure should be measured immediately before the surgery and monitored at approximately 1-hour intervals for 2 to 3 hours after treatment. The majority of patients who develop a posttreatment spike in intraocular pressure do so within the first hour (Weinreb et al 1983). Elevation of intraocular pressure to significantly higher levels than noted preoperatively occurs in 25% to 50% of treated patients (Goldstick and Weinreb 1989). If no pressure spike occurs within 2 to 3 hours, the risk falls to nearly zero. A 24-hour check of intraocular pressure is desirable, however, because a few patients may not show the rise until many hours after treatment and it may persist at high levels for days thereafter if untreated. The risk of immediate rise in intraocular pressure after laser surgery is less with 180° than with 360° treatment (Goldstick and Weinreb 1989).

The preoperative assessment should include estimating the risk of aggravating optic nerve injury by a transient rise in intraocular pressure postoperatively. Planning should include the possibility of needing to vigorously treat a postoperative spike. A very small percentage of patients have persisting elevation of intraocular pressure after ALT and may require urgent filtering surgery. No correlation has been demonstrated between the immediate postoperative spike in intraocular pressure and the long-term success or failure

of the procedure. In patients with advanced optic nerve injury, it may be prudent to treat only 180° in addition to prophylactic use of pressure-lowering medications.

Besides reapplication of apraclonidine or other topical or systemic agents to prevent postoperative pressure spikes (beta blockers, miotics, carbonic anhydrase inhibitors), regular use of antiglaucoma medications should be continued until the effect of the laser can be assessed over 4 to 6 weeks. Topical steroids are occasionally necessary to minimize immediate postoperative inflammation, but usually for no more than a week.

Routine followup, assuming no sharp rise in intraocular pressure, can be done at 24 hours and at 3 and 6 weeks with continued use of regular medications.

COMPLICATIONS

Bleeding from Schlemm's canal may occasionally occur during ALT, but rapidly stops with continued compression by the goniolens. Microhyphema may aggravate the elevation of intraocular pressure in the immediate postoperative period.

Besides the immediate or delayed rise in intraocular pressure, complications noted after ALT have included corneal burns, persistent inflammation (which has rarely been severe), pupil or iris distortion and dysfunction, and formation of focal peripheral anterior synechiae (PAS) corresponding to the burn locations. PAS formation probably indicates that the burns were too intense. Avoiding treatment of the posterior meshwork may decrease the risk of PAS formation. Pigment dispersion or irregularity within the meshwork is common after ALT in the areas treated, but the typical lesions noted during treatment will have faded by 24 to 48 hours later. In extremely rare instances, possibly associated with unrecognized spikes in intraocular pressure, iris infarction and hemorrhage, central retinal vessel occlusions, or loss of additional vision including "snuff-out" has been reported (Hoskins et al 1983).

An additional possible complication of ALT, in patients with narrow anterior chamber angles, is acceleration of progressive closure of the angle. When confronted by an unexpectedly narrow angle during attempted ALT, the surgeon may reasonably elect to defer the procedure, consider iridoplasty as a mechanism to open the angle, or reconsider the diagnosis and possible need for iridectomy as an alternative form of treatment.

14-6
DELAY AND RE-TREATMENT

Rational use of ALT would seem to include allowing sufficient time postoperatively (4 to 6 weeks) to assess the effect before proceeding with filtration surgery. In some patients, with badly damaged discs and high intraocular pressure, laser therapy may adversely delay more effective surgical therapy. Prompt surgery in patients with advanced optic nerve injury and high levels of intraocular pressure may be preferable to ALT.

Treatment of the second 180° may be effective in some patients who fail to respond to the initial treatment. Re-treatment of previously treated areas has yielded less than a 50% success rate, decreasing to only 14% after 1 year with increased risk of complications (Richter et al 1987).

14-7
PATHOPHYSIOLOGY

The mechanism by which ALT lowers intraocular pressure is not known, although an immediate "mechanical" effect on the meshwork is widely accepted (Wise and Witter 1979). Besides the immediate thermal effect of the burns on surrounding tissues, apparently including tightening of the meshwork (circumferential shortening), there may be a long-term metabolic effect (Van Buskirk et al 1984). Certainly, the application of laser burns produces focal tissue necrosis and stimulates repair processes, probably including endothelial migration into the injured areas. Excessive burns of the angle structures and adjacent ciliary body can produce secondary glaucoma in the monkey eye, including endothelial and Descemet's membrane extension over the damaged meshwork (Minckler et al 1987).

14-8

SUMMARY

Argon laser trabeculoplasty has been a valuable addition to therapy in open-angle glaucoma. However, its effects are limited in duration and it is seldom an adequate substitute for topical medications. ALT remains controversial as an alternative to medication as primary therapy in open-angle glaucoma. ALT is particularly effective in older patients whose glaucoma is associated with pseudoexfoliation and pigmentary dispersion. Pretreatment of eyes with apraclonidine has been shown to dramatically reduce the risk of transient high intraocular pressure following ALT.

BIBLIOGRAPHY

Glaucoma Laser Trial Research Group: the Glaucoma Laser Trial (GLT). *Ophthalmology* 1990;**97**:1404–1413.

Goldstick BJ, Weinreb RN: Laser treatment in open-angle glaucoma. In: Ritch R, Shields MB, Krupin T, eds: *The Glaucomas*. St Louis: CV Mosby Co; 1989:605–620.

Hoskins HD, Hetherington J, Minckler DS, et al: Complications of laser trabeculoplasty. *Ophthalmology* 1983;**90**:796–799.

Minckler DS, Shammas A, Wilcox M, et al: Experimental studies of aqueous filtration using the Molteno implant. *Trans Am Ophthalmol Soc* 1987;**85**:368–392.

Richter CU, Shingleton BJ, Bellows AR, et al: Retreatment with argon laser trabeculoplasty. *Ophthalmology* 1987;**94**:1085–1089.

Robin AL, Pollack IP, House B, et al: Effects of ALO 2145 on intraocular pressure following argon laser trabeculoplasty. *Arch Ophthalmol* 1987;**105**:646–650.

Schultz JS, Werner EB, Krupin T, et al: Intraocular pressure and visual field defects after argon laser trabeculoplasty in chronic open-angle glaucoma. *Ophthalmology* 1987;**94**:553–557.

Schwartz AL, Love DC, Schwartz MA: Long-term follow-up of argon laser trabeculoplasty for uncontrolled open-angle glaucoma. *Arch Ophthalmol* 1985:**103**:1482–1484.

Van Buskirk EM, Pone V, Rosenquist RC, et al: Argon laser trabeculoplasty: studies of mechanism of action. *Ophthalmology* 1984;**91**: 1005–1009.

Weinreb RN, Ruderman J, Juster R, et al: Immediate intraocular pressure response to argon laser trabeculoplasty. *Am J Ophthalmol* 1983; **95**:279–286.

Wise JB, Witter SL: Argon laser therapy for open-angle glaucoma. *Arch Ophthalmol* 1979;**97**: 319–322.

Commentary

Robert N. Weinreb, MD

Dr Minckler raises a number of issues worthy of discussion:

1. I regard argon laser trabeculoplasty to be a surgical procedure, and therefore consider treating only one eye during a session. I have examined 5 patients who received bilateral treatment in one session and who had serious sequelae in both eyes. One 62-year-old man who had bilateral laser trabeculoplasty experienced a serious rise in intraocular pressure with concomitant iritis in both eyes that could not be medically controlled. Admittedly, such events are rare, but I see no reason to treat two eyes during one session.

2. For several years, I have performed laser trabeculoplasty by treating over 360° using 80 to 100 laser burns in one treatment session. Unquestionably, the incidence and magnitude of intraocular pressure rise following laser trabeculoplasty is less when half as many laser burns are administered over 180°. However, by monitoring intraocular pressure for 2 to 3 hours postoperatively, as suggested by Dr Minckler, the surgeon can recognize a rise in intraocular pressure and treat it appropriately. During the past few years, the use of apraclonidine has been particularly beneficial in this regard. Although I do not employ it routinely as preoperative medication, I do administer apraclonidine 1 hour before and after argon laser trabeculoplasty in eyes with advanced optic nerve injury. I then observe the patient until intraocular pressure is noted to decrease.

3. I have found the Ritch trabeculoplasty lens to be helpful in this procedure. It has two basic mirrors: one inclined at an angle of 59°, which allows a face-on view of the inferior half of the angle; and one inclined at 64°, which allows a similar view of the superior half of the angle. The Ritch lens has two additional mirrors inclined at the same angle with superimposed planoconvex buttons that produce ×1.4 magnification.

Commentary

E. Michael Van Buskirk, MD

Argon laser trabeculoplasty has become a standard technique for treating open-angle varieties of adult glaucoma, such as primary open-angle, pseudoexfoliation, and pigmentary glaucomas. As Dr Minckler indicates, the procedure does not work well for inflammatory glaucoma. In fact, it may irreversibly elevate intraocular pressure. The principal issues for argon laser trabeculoplasty now concern whether it should be used early or late and whether or not it can be repeated. My experience has been that patients who have had a lasting (1 year or longer), unquestionably positive effect but that ultimately diminishes respond favorably to subsequent laser trabeculoplasty. In contrast, patients who have had an equivocal response to the initial laser therapy do not respond favorably to subsequent treatment.

The technique of laser trabeculoplasty is largely empiric, based on the experience of others with successful results. However, variations in technique have not produced significant changes in results, except with markedly reduced power or number of burns. I prefer to treat 180° because many patients achieve a satisfactory effect and the opposite 180° can be preserved for later treatment if necessary.

The surgeon should be well familiar with the gonioscopic landmarks of the particular eye to be treated before undertaking laser trabeculoplasty. It is worthwhile to reassess the chamber angle at the laser slit lamp in each patient before starting the procedure.

CHAPTER 15

Laser Iridotomy

Richard A. Lewis, MD

The surgical treatment of angle-closure glaucoma due to pupillary block has been advanced with the widespread availability of the argon and Nd:YAG lasers. These lasers permit the surgeon to establish an iridotomy inside the eye without incising the globe. The argon laser creates the iridotomy through a thermal effect that depends on heat absorption by pigmented tissues, while the Nd:YAG laser acts through an electromechanical photodisruption independent of pigmentation.

15-1

INDICATIONS

Laser iridotomy is indicated in the treatment of acute and chronic angle-closure glaucoma, combined-mechanism glaucoma, pseudophakic and aphakic pupillary-block glaucoma, and incomplete surgical iridectomy. Difficulties can be expected in certain clinical settings, including uncooperative patients or those with nausea or vomiting. In addition, ocular disease associated with a shallow anterior chamber, corneal edema or opacification, inflammation, middilated pupils, or thick irides may present problems for the laser surgeon.

15-2

SURGICAL TECHNIQUE

The patient is premedicated with a topical anesthetic. Retrobulbar anesthesia is usually unnecessary for laser iridotomy. However, if the patient has nausea, vomiting, and ocular pain associated with marked elevation of intraocular pressure from acute angle-closure glaucoma, a retrobulbar anesthetic block quickly alleviates these symptoms. It also aids in the administration of oral agents to lower intraocular pressure and elicits greater patient cooperation during the laser surgery.

Pretreating the patient with a miotic agent such as pilocarpine is advantageous. The miotic pupil provides greater iris surface area for treatment and minimizes the chance of errant laser energy causing retinal injury. Prophylactic hypotensive therapy is recommended because 30% of patients develop elevated intraocular pressure after laser iridotomy. Pretreatment with carbonic anhydrase inhibitors or a topical beta-adrenergic blocking agent may prevent a post-laser spike in intraocular pressure, but the drug of choice is apraclonidine, an alpha-2 agonist. This topical medication is given an hour prior to the laser surgery, and a second drop is applied at the completion of the treatment. In addition to preventing the post-laser pressure spike, apraclonidine is a vasoconstrictor and may aid in limiting the amount of iris bleeding when the Nd:YAG laser is used.

Proper positioning of the patient at the slit lamp is very important. Both the surgeon and the patient must be comfortable; otherwise, the procedure may take much more time. The patient should be seated comfortably, with the chin in the chin rest and the level of the eye adjusted to the indicated level of the instrument.

Application of the Abraham laser iridotomy lens greatly facilitates laser iris surgery. The Abraham lens has a high-power planoconvex button affixed to the anterior surface of a contact lens and is applied with methylcellulose solution. The planoconvex button helps focus and magnify the laser energy. Alternative lenses have been described, including the Wise lens, which provides a higher power density at the tissue site, but causes greater image distortion due to higher magnification; and the Lasag CGI lens. The lenses aid in lid retraction, control of eye movement, and prevention of corneal burns by acting as heat sinks.

The procedure is best executed with high magnification through the ×40 power of the slit lamp plus the iridotomy lens. After the surgeon has localized a thin area or crypt on the superior iris, it is critical to focus on the specific surface site selected prior to each application. The superior aspect of the iris is preferred for treatment because it will be concealed by the upper lid and, thus, reduce postoperative glare. The surgeon should avoid treating through an arcus senilis because it will obscure visualization of the iridotomy site and defocus the laser energy. The surgeon should aim away from the posterior pole and direct the energy to the peripheral iris.

With the argon laser, a 50-micron spot size, 0.1- to 0.2-second duration, and 600 to 1200 mW of power are customary, although no consensus exists on the specific laser parameters and a variety of techniques have been described. The most popular include one or a combination of the following:

1. Preparatory burns to put the iris on stretch.

2. A "chipping" approach, using multiple brief (0.02 second) exposures.

3. A two-step procedure: (a) The initial application uses high power (1500 mW) and long duration (0.5 second) to achieve a gas bubble on the iris surface; the bubble acts as an additional magnifying source to refocus the laser energy at the base of the iridotomy site. (b) Then the power is reduced to 1000 mW and the duration to 0.05 second to penetrate the bubble and the iris pigment epithelium.

A successful outcome depends on different variables, including iris color and thickness, corneal clarity, and, most important, an experienced surgeon. If after the initial laser exposures a site appears to show little or no response or if iris "charring" becomes apparent, the surgeon should consider an alternative site and different energy levels.

Specific recommendations for the Nd:YAG laser depend to a great extent on the particular laser. In general, the energy settings range from 2 to 6 mJ with a burst of 1 to 6 pulses per application. The number of applications necessary to complete the iridotomy with the Nd:YAG laser is often fewer than 10. Although higher energy levels may ensure greater likelihood of penetration, they also increase the risk of bleeding.

15-3

RESULTS

The end point of treatment for both laser modalities is a patent iridotomy. This can be recognized by a clear iris transillumination defect and visualization of the lens capsule through the iris. Another useful sign of penetration through the iris pigmented epithelium is the pigment epithelial storm (smokestack effect). The ultimate size of the iridotomy is less important than the clear demonstration of patency. Although deepening of the anterior chamber may be noted during the procedure, alleviation of angle-closure glaucoma depends on the post-laser gonioscopic appearance of the angle structures.

Closure or "healing" of the defect may occur, although it is unusual with the Nd:YAG laser. It is advantageous to perform multiple iridotomies if any possibility of late closure exists. This is most likely to occur in the presence of rubeosis iridis, chronic uveitis, and aphakic or pseudophakic pupillary block. At times, combining the cauterizing effect of the argon laser with that of the Nd:YAG laser is advantageous in patients with iris vascularity.

Although both the argon and the Nd:YAG lasers have high success rates in achieving patent iridotomies, there are differences. The Nd:YAG laser requires less total energy and fewer pulses, and it penetrates regardless of iris color. As a result, it has no effect on pupil shape. Furthermore, the Nd:YAG laser is portable and, thus, allows greater access to more patients. The greatest disadvantage of the Nd:YAG is the risk of bleeding, which occurs in 45% of patients but is usually transient and clears spontaneously. If bleeding occurs, it may be stopped by applying pressure to the eye through the contact lens. The absence of bleeding during iridotomy is an important advantage of the argon laser. Thus, it is particularly valuable in patients with engorged iris vessels or rubeosis and in patients taking anticoagulants. Over the long term, there is no significant difference in safety or efficacy between the two lasers.

POSTOPERATIVE CARE

After laser surgery, the patient should be examined during the subsequent 3 hours and again within the next week. It is important to measure intraocular pressure, anterior chamber reaction, and patency of the iridotomy. In patients with angle closure, it is also important to re-examine the angle structures with a gonioprism.

POSTOPERATIVE COMPLICATIONS

Both argon and Nd:YAG lasers share similar postoperative complications. A transient iritis due to pigment debris and inflammatory mediators is found in virtually every patient. Topical steroids are occasionally necessary, but usually for no more than a week. A post-laser increase in intraocular pressure of greater than 10 mm Hg occurs in 30% of patients. It is important to pretreat with hypotensive agents and check pressure during the first 1 to 3 hours after completion of the iridotomy. Focal corneal opacities may be noted, particularly in eyes with a shallow chamber. This problem can be minimized with the Abraham iridotomy lens and sharp focus. If a corneal opacity develops, the surgeon should select another location because the opacity will diminish the amount of laser energy transmitted. Focal, nonprogressive lens opacities have also been documented in 35% of patients treated with the argon laser, but they are not associated with visual loss. Inadvertent retinal burns, if localized to the macular area, may induce visual loss, especially after penetration of the iris. It is important to direct the laser energy away from the posterior pole and toward the peripheral retina.

15-6

SUMMARY

Laser iridotomy has profoundly affected the treatment of angle-closure glaucoma and has largely replaced incisional surgical iridectomy. However, the relative ease of laser iridotomy does not supplant good clinical judgment in regard to indications, technique, and postoperative care.

BIBLIOGRAPHY

Brown RH, Lynch MG: Laser peripheral iridotomy for pupillary-block glaucoma. *Ophthalmology* 1989(suppl, pt 2):218–228.

Kolker AE: Techniques of argon laser iridectomy. *Trans Am Ophthalmol Soc.* 1984;**82**:302–306.

Simmons RJ, Savage JA, Belcher CD, et al: Usual and unusual uses of the laser in glaucoma. In: *Symposium on the Laser in Ophthalmology and Glaucoma Update. Trans New Orleans Acad Ophthalmol.* St Louis: CV Mosby Co; 1985:154–175.

Commentary

Donald S. Minckler, MD

This chapter nicely summarizes the performance of iridotomies with either argon or Nd:YAG lasers. The importance of using a condensing lens such as the Abraham with the argon laser or an alternative iris plane lens such as that manufactured by Lasag cannot be overemphasized.

These lenses make iridectomy by laser far more practical and safe than without such lenses. When using the argon laser, the surgeon must closely watch the depth of the anterior chamber and avoid treating gas bubbles that contact the endothelium. Significant endothelial burns may result if the gas bubble is in contact with the endothelium. A pigment epithelial storm (smokestack effect) is a good sign of penetration of the pigment epithelium with the argon laser. With either argon or Nd:YAG lasers, pupillary block should be relieved when penetration and significant deepening of the chamber occur.

In patients with inflammatory seclusion of the pupil, iridectomy or iridotomy may be best performed incisionally rather than with a laser. Laser iridotomies are virtually always relatively small and far more likely to close in the days to weeks following the procedure than is an incisional iridectomy in an inflamed eye.

Combining the cautery effect of the argon laser and the speed of the Nd:YAG laser may sometimes be advantageous, especially in thick brown irides. The argon laser may be used initially to flatten and cauterize the iris stroma, and the Nd:YAG laser subsequently at the same site to effect an opening. Nd:YAG laser energy should be reduced from that usually utilized because the previous use of the argon laser may enhance the effect of the Nd:YAG laser.

Commentary

Robert N. Weinreb, MD

The selection of either the argon or the Nd:YAG laser for creating an iridotomy is often based on convenience. In other words, the surgeon may choose to use either a laser that is already in the office or one that is readily available. Because there should be little difficulty in creating a patent iridotomy with either laser and since the ultimate success is apparently similar, only a few factors can otherwise guide a surgeon in choosing a particular laser.

Although I have immediate access to both lasers, I use the Nd:YAG laser in most cases. With fewer laser applications than with the argon laser, the procedure is better tolerated by patients. Further, it is extremely unusual to have to repeat an iridotomy because of closure of a previously patent iridotomy. Although 50% of the patients I have treated experienced a small amount of bleeding, this has not posed a problem. Applying pressure to the contact lens is most often sufficient to stop the bleeding. Recently, I have treated patients 1 hour prior to Nd:YAG iridotomy with apraclonidine 1% to reduce bleeding. However, with patients who have been treated with anticoagulants or who have uveitis or iris neovascularization, I use the argon laser because it is less likely to be associated with bleeding.

CHAPTER 16

Other Uses of the Laser

J. Rigby Slight, MD

By taking advantage of the photocoagulation effects of the argon laser and the photodisruptive effects of the Nd:YAG laser, the surgeon will find a number of other uses of the laser in glaucoma besides laser trabeculoplasty and iridotomy.

16-1

PERIPHERAL IRIDOPLASTY

In laser peripheral iridoplasty (also known as gonioplasty), the configuration of the iris is changed by placing a series of argon laser burns on the iris surface. These photocoagulative burns cause the iris tissue to contract. When placed along the peripheral roll of the iris, the burns can be used to widen a narrow angle (Figure 16-1). This is a useful adjunct in argon laser trabeculoplasty when a superimposed anatomic narrow angle interferes with the placement of trabeculoplasty burns on the trabecular meshwork.

One method of opening the angle with iridoplasty is accomplished by directing the laser beam onto the peripheral roll of the iris through the gonioscopy mirror of a Goldmann 3-mirror lens, using a spot size

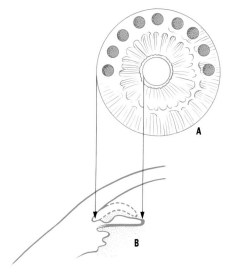

Figure 16-1 *Peripheral iridoplasty. Large, low-power, long-duration argon laser burns cause the peripheral iris to shrink and contract to open a narrow angle if synechiae are not present. (A) Anterior view. (B) Cross section.*

of 200 microns, an exposure time of 0.2 second, and starting with a power setting of 200 mW. If the tissue reaction is insufficient to widen the angle or cause contraction, the power setting is gradually increased until the desired tissue alteration is accomplished. This method is most useful when 90° or less of the superior angle is narrow and requires treatment.

When a larger portion of the angle needs to be opened, it is easier and takes less time to enlarge the spot size to 500 microns, increase the time to 0.5 second, and titrate the power (depending on the tissue reaction) starting at 200 mW. With this technique, the laser beam is directed through the central portion of the Goldmann lens directly onto the peripheral iris.

In addition to widening the angle in patients undergoing argon laser trabeculoplasty, iridoplasty can also be used as an adjunct in the treatment of certain patients with narrow-angle glaucoma. For example, it can be used to increase the space between the iris and the corneal endothelium in patients for whom laser iridotomy would cause endothelial damage because of the close proximity of the iris and cornea. Once the space has been increased, laser iridotomy can be performed. Peripheral iridoplasty may be beneficial also in treating patients with nanophthalmos to prevent or delay total angle closure

because laser peripheral iridotomy is not helpful. Further, iridoplasty may be useful in the treatment of the plateau iris syndrome, in which the angle remains occludable despite a patent peripheral iridotomy. The role of iridoplasty in delaying or preventing gradual angle closure in chronic narrow-angle-closure glaucoma remains to be established.

16-2

PUPILLOPLASTY, PHOTOMYDRIASIS, AND SPHINCTEROTOMY

Pupilloplasty and photomydriasis are procedures like iridoplasty in which the photocoagulative effects of the argon laser are used to shrink the tissue of the iris and to alter the shape of the pupil.

In pupillary-block glaucoma, a series of laser burns can be placed along one sector of the iris close to the collarette, causing the pupil to peak sufficiently to release the pupillary block and allow the anterior chamber to deepen. Once the chamber has deepened and inflammation of the cornea and anterior segment has cleared, the surgeon can proceed to a definitive peripheral iridotomy with ease and safety. Pupilloplasty can be accomplished using a 200-micron spot size for 0.2 second starting at a power setting of 200 mW and increasing the power until the appropriate tissue reaction is apparent. Pupilloplasty is especially useful in pupillary-block glaucoma when there is blockage between an anterior chamber intraocular lens and the iris, and the peripheral iris is bowed so far forward that it is in apposition with the peripheral cornea.

Photomydriasis is used to enlarge the pupillary aperture in patients on long-term miotic therapy in whom the small pupil significantly interferes with their vision (therapeutic) or in those in whom a miotic pupil precludes examination of the posterior segment (diagnostic). A series of 500-micron burns placed in double concentric rings in the middle portion of the iris often can enlarge a 1-mm pupil to 4 mm (Figure 16-2). As in iridoplasty, a duration of 0.5 second with a power setting of 200 mW is a good starting point. Prior to performing therapeutic photomydriasis, the surgeon should demonstrate and document a subjective improvement in the patient's vision following the use of mydriatics. If this is not done, the likelihood is that the patient will have a disappointing visual result.

Pupillary enlargement can also be accomplished by argon or Nd:YAG laser sphincterotomy. This can be accomplished by making a radial cut across the sphincter fibers with a lens that highly focuses and increases the power density of the laser on the iris, such as the Abraham iridectomy lens or the Wise iridotomy-sphincterotomy lens. A radial incision is made across the sphincter with the argon laser, using exposures of 0.01 and 0.02 second, a 50-micron spot size, and a power level between 800 and 1500 mW. Most sphincterotomies may be completed with 200 to 400 laser burns. The Nd:YAG laser can also be used for sphincterotomy in aphakic eyes using one of the condensing lenses and multiple low-energy single pulses between 1 and 4 mJ.

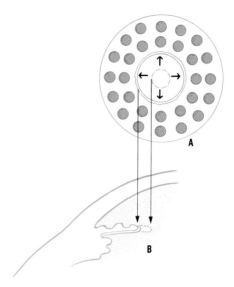

Figure 16-2 *Photomydriasis. A double row of large, low-power, long-duration argon laser burns causes contraction of the iris and enlargement of the pupil. (A) Anterior view. (B) Cross section.*

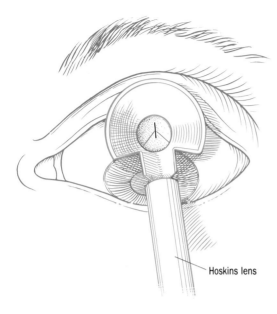
Hoskins lens

Figure 16-3 *Trabeculectomy flap suture release. The transparent Hoskins lens button compresses and blanches the underlying conjunctiva, improving the visualization of the suture and making it easier to cut the suture with the argon laser.*

16-3

RELEASE OF A TRABECULECTOMY FLAP SUTURE

The incidence of flat chambers associated with trabeculectomy can be reduced by suturing the scleral flap more tightly into the scleral bed. However, when the flap is sutured firmly, intraocular pressure tends to become elevated in the early postoperative period because of reduced aqueous flow. The flow may be increased by cutting one or more of the sutures with the argon laser. Because the conjunctival incision has begun to heal, resistance to flow is increased and, subsequently, there is less chance of a flat chamber at this stage in the postoperative period.

The Hoskins nylon suture lens is very helpful in cutting the suture because it can be used to compress the overlying conjunctiva and blood vessels, thereby enhancing visualization of the suture (Figure 16-3). The flange on the lens holds the upper lid out of the way. As an alternative, the central portion of the Zeiss 4-mirror lens can be used to release the trabeculectomy flap suture. The suture can be cut using a spot size of 100 microns for 0.1 second with a power setting between 500 mW and 1.0 W on the argon laser. A krypton red laser can also be used to cut the flap suture, particularly when the suture is partly obscured by the presence of subconjunctival hemorrhage.

16-4

GONIOPHOTOCOAGULATION

Neovascular glaucoma is among the most refractory forms of glaucoma to either medical or surgical therapy. The neovascularization must be halted before irreversible angle changes have taken place and chronic angle-closure glaucoma has ensued. The stimulus for neovascularization can be curtailed by ablating the ischemic retina with panretinal photocoagulation, cryoablation, or endophotocoagulation during vitreous surgery. In certain patients, there is a period of time when intraocular pressure is elevated secondary to a fibrovascular membrane in the angle and the stimulus for neovascularization has not totally regressed despite adequate panretinal photocoagulation. In these selected patients, the intraocular pressure elevation can sometimes be transiently controlled and angle closure delayed by directly photocoagulating angle vessels and peripheral iris vessels using a spot size of 100 to 200 microns for 0.2 second with a power setting between 200 and 700 mW (Figure 16-4). Blanching or obliterating the vessels is the end point and often requires up to several hundred applications divided over several sessions. This procedure is of little or no benefit except as a temporary measure in patients who are receiving or have received sufficient ablation to the ischemic retina.

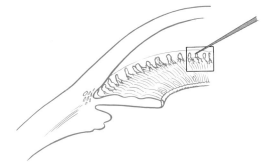

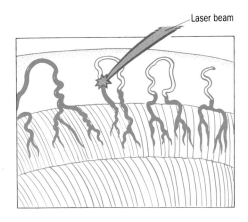

Laser beam

Figure 16-4 *Goniophotocoagulation. Argon laser burns directed onto the new angle vessels coagulate and temporarily close the vessels while awaiting the results of retinal ablation measures.*

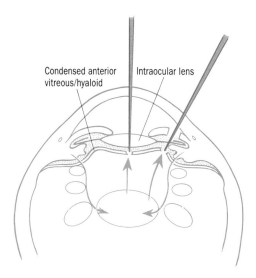

Condensed anterior vitreous/hyaloid   Intraocular lens

Figure 16-5 *Aphakic/pseudophakic malignant glaucoma. The condensed anterior vitreous/hyaloid acts like a one-way valve, allowing aqueous to flow posteriorly but not anteriorly. The Nd:YAG laser can disrupt this condensation either through a peripheral iridectomy if present or directly through the intraocular lens, releasing the trapped aqueous to come forward.*

16-5

PHOTOCOAGULATION FOR MALIGNANT GLAUCOMA

In malignant glaucoma, aqueous humor flow is misdirected posteriorly within or behind the vitreous, leading to secondary angle-closure glaucoma. The phakic eyes in which this occurs tend to have a close approximation between the ciliary body and the lens, creating a ciliolenticular block that directs the aqueous posteriorly. In patients who have not responded to medical therapy, it is sometimes possible to disrupt the block by photocoagulating the ciliary processes when they are visible through an iridectomy. The shrinkage of the ciliary processes frees the aqueous trapped posteriorly, allowing forward flow with deepening of the anterior chamber and opening of the closed angle. Shrinkage of the ciliary processes can usually be accomplished by directing an argon laser beam through the gonioscopy mirror using a spot size of 200 microns for 0.2 second and a power setting between 400 and 800 mW.

A similar problem can occur in aphakic or pseudophakic eyes where a ciliovitreal or ciliovitreopseudophakic block seems to cause a misdirection of aqueous humor flow posteriorly. In these patients, the anterior hyaloid membrane of the vitreous acts as a barrier blocking the forward movement of the aqueous into the anterior segment. It is possible to release this block by disrupting the anterior hyaloid and anterior vitreous with the Nd:YAG laser, creating a passageway between the anterior segment and the aqueous trapped posteriorly (Figure 16-5). The settings will differ depending on the specific laser employed.

16-6

SUMMARY

A number of other uses of the laser for glaucoma in addition to laser trabeculoplasty and iridotomy are the result of matching the mode of action of the laser to the tissue type or substance that needs to be altered to obtain the desired effect. The argon laser requires pigment to absorb the laser energy and is most effective in altering the shape of the iris and ciliary body, cutting sutures, coagulating blood vessels, and penetrating pigmented membranes. The Nd:YAG laser, on the other hand, does not require the presence of pigment and is useful in disrupting nonpigmented membranes and the vitreous. Attention to these principles enhances the multiple other uses of the laser in glaucoma.

BIBLIOGRAPHY

Herschler J: Laser shrinkage of the ciliary processes: a treatment for malignant (ciliary block) glaucoma. *Ophthalmology* 1980;**87**: 1155–1158.

Hoskins HD Jr, Migliazzo C: Management of failing filtering blebs with the argon laser. *Ophthalmic Surg* 1984;**15**:731–733.

Ritch R: Argon laser treatment of medically unresponsive attacks of angle closure glaucoma. *Am J Ophthalmol* 1982;**94**:197–204.

Simmons RJ, Deppermann SR, Dueker DK: The role of goniophotocoagulation in neovascularization of the anterior chamber angle. *Ophthalmology* 1980;**87**:79–82.

Wise JB: Iris sphincterotomy, iridotomy and synechiotomy by linear incision with the argon laser. *Ophthalmology* 1985;**92**:641–645.

Commentary

E. Michael Van Buskirk, MD

Dr Slight has presented a "menu" of other uses of the laser in the management of glaucoma patients—uses other than iridotomy, trabeculoplasty, and ciliodestruction. Many of these procedures are of temporary use to facilitate more definitive approaches. All of these procedures involve cutting or stretching tissue with photocoagulative or photodisruptive lasers.

When using an argon or other photocoagulating laser, the surgeon should remember the general principles. A narrow, focal, high-energy, short-duration burn tends to cut, while a longer, broader, lower-energy burn is more likely to produce tissue shrinkage without cutting. Thus, if stretching of the iris is wanted—

as with iridoplasty or pupilloplasty—the larger-diameter, lower-power burns should be used.

Gonioplasty or peripheral iridoplasty for widening a narrow angle to facilitate argon laser trabeculoplasty is occasionally useful, but should be approached with caution. Patients with combined angle-closure and open-angle glaucoma carry a more guarded prognosis for successful laser trabeculoplasty, even when it is technically possible to perform the trabeculoplasty or even if the patients have had a laser iridotomy to eliminate the pupillary-block component of their glaucoma. Gonioplasty may make it technically feasible to treat the trabecular meshwork, but may create peripheral iris inflammation leading to peripheral anterior synechiae. Many of these patients ultimately require trabeculectomy. Often, the trabecular meshwork can be treated even in the presence of a narrow but open angle by using the intermediate mirror of the three-mirror Goldmann lens and asking the patient to look toward the mirror. This permits visualization over the peripheral iris roll without photocoagulating the iris periphery.

My experience with photomydriasis is that it has been temporary, not permanent. This makes it useful for breaking an attack of pupillary block and deepening the chamber to allow a more definitive laser iridotomy, as Dr Slight mentions. I have usually found that attempts to dilate the pupil permanently are unsuccessful.

As Dr Slight mentions, goniophotocoagulation for neovascular glaucoma should be used only to supplement the more definitive retinal ablative procedures. However, a less destructive method of treatment can be applied to eyes in which neovascular fronds are just beginning to arborize in the trabecular meshwork. The fronds are evident clinically as a vascular trunk extending from the root of the iris over the scleral spur and then arborizing into the trabecular meshwork. These feeder trunks can be coagulated as they cross the scleral spur to devitalize the entire arborization. I agree with Dr Slight that this procedure is usually of little value, except in those patients who have already had a retinal ablative procedure.

In the management of aphakic or pseudophakic malignant glaucoma, disruption of the posterior as well as anterior hyaloid is sometimes necessary to allow the posteriorly entrapped aqueous humor access to the anterior chamber.

Photocoagulation of an unwanted cyclodialysis cleft in the management of hypotony also deserves mention. Burns with a spot size of 200 to 500 microns can be applied within the cyclodialysis cleft to create sufficient inflammation to allow closure of the cleft. Following the procedure, the patient should be treated with a cycloplegic to achieve maximal narrowing of the space.

Commentary

Richard A. Lewis, MD

The laser has continued to evolve in its application to the diagnosis and treatment of glaucoma. In patients with epithelial downgrowth, the argon laser can be used to identify the extent of the downgrowth on the iris. With a low power of between 200 and 400 mW and a spot size of 50 to 100 microns, the leading edge of the epithelium can be identified by placing laser applications to the anterior surface of the iris. Epithelium turns white, while iris tissue does not.

Another use of the laser involves the shrinkage of conjunctival blebs. The argon laser can be used to contract tissue on the superficial surface of the bleb. This is particularly useful in moderately elevated blebs overlying the cornea. With low power and a large spot size, conjunctival shrinkage can be identified. Applying a dye to the surface of the eye allows for greater uptake of laser energy. In addition, abrading the surface of the bleb is sometimes useful so that the laser will cause greater contraction of tissue.

The Nd:YAG laser has also been used to enlarge pupillary size in distorted or miotic pupils. This use should be limited to aphakic or pseudophakic eyes. The Nd:YAG laser can cut or enlarge the pupil by direct application to the anterior iris surface.

CHAPTER 17

Cyclocryotherapy

E. Michael Van Buskirk, MD

Procedures that injure or destroy the ciliary processes as a method of inhibiting aqueous humor formation have been used for the past half-century to treat refractory glaucoma. Cyclodestructive techniques employing cautery were generally replaced by cryotherapy in the early 1960s. More recently, laser and ultrasound therapy have been used to achieve the same end.

17-1

INDICATIONS

Cyclocryotherapy and other cyclodestructive procedures are generally reserved for patients who have a poor prognosis for filtration surgery, such as those who have had multiple previous intraocular operations, have severely scarred conjunctiva, or have chronic ocular inflammation or neovascularization. Cyclodestructive procedures may also be ideal for pain reduction in those patients with limited visual potential. In addition, cyclocryotherapy predictably reduces intraocular pressure to a safe zone in a high percentage of pa-

tients with aphakic open-angle glaucoma. Unpredictable loss of visual acuity from macular edema, however, diminishes its appeal for patients with good vision. The procedure is easily and rapidly performed in an outpatient setting with only retrobulbar anesthesia.

17-2

SURGICAL TECHNIQUE

The goal of the procedure is to destroy focally the ciliary process epithelium by freezing with a cryoprobe through the intact conjunctiva, sclera, and ciliary muscle. The extent of the area treated can be adjusted to the amount of hypotensive response required, but usually 120° to 180° of cyclodestruction is required. Treating the entire circumference of the ciliary body in one session is associated with a high incidence of phthisis bulbi and probably should be avoided.

Technically, 6 clock hours (180°) should be treated initially, with additional treatments if the hypotensive response is insufficient. As few as 3 or 4 clock hours of treatment produce less pain and inflammation and may be sufficient for patients

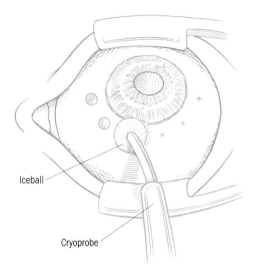

Figure 17-1 *Cryoprobe for glaucoma cyclocryotherapy with tip 2.0 mm posterior to the limbus.*

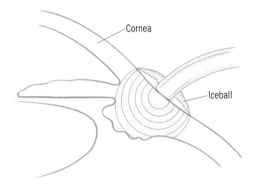

Figure 17-2 *Cross-sectional view of cryoprobe 2 mm behind the limbus showing scleral uveal iceball.*

with some functioning outflow and mild intraocular pressure elevation.

Anxious patients may be given mild oral sedation such as 5 mg diazepam 30 minutes prior to the procedure, but no preoperative sedation is usually necessary. Retrobulbar anesthetic 3 cc is administered, usually with a 50:50 mixture of 0.75% bupivacaine and 2% lidocaine. A glaucoma cryoprobe with a head 3.5 mm in diameter with nitrous oxide should be used with the cryotherapy apparatus to achieve $-80°C$ at the probe tip. The probe should be applied warm to the eye 2 mm posterior to the limbus, and freezing applied for 50 to 60 seconds (Figure 17-1). An iceball 7 to 10 mm in diameter will be visible emanating at the probe tip (Figure 17-2). After 60 seconds of freez-

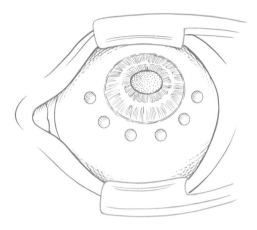

Figure 17-3 *Immediate postoperative view showing sites of six cryotherapy applications over 180°.*

ing, an assistant irrigates the probe and conjunctiva with balanced salt solution to prevent unduly prolonged freezing and to permit nontraumatic removal of the probe. A total of 5 to 6 contiguous applications should be applied over 180° of the global circumference depending on the lateral diameter of the iceballs (Figure 17-3).

At the end of the procedure, a subconjunctival injection of 3 mg betamethasone suspension greatly diminishes postoperative inflammation and pain. Patients who exhibit significant postoperative pain require oral narcotic analgesics such as codeine 60 mg. Frequent topical prednisolone further diminishes postoperative inflammation.

17-3

COMPLICATIONS

Cyclocryotherapy invariably causes some postoperative uveitis, which usually diminishes over several weeks. Severe pain, associated with inflammation, may ensue. Topical cycloplegics or corticosterioids diminish pain as well as inflammation. Severe chemosis may require ocular lubricants. Occasionally, a chronic smoldering inflammation persists that can be associated with cystoid macular edema, ciliochoroidal detachments, and, rarely, phthisis bulbi. Confining therapy to 180° markedly reduces the risk of these complications, but because they are possible, the procedure is seldom used for patients whose visual potential is greater than 20/200 (6/60).

17-4

SUMMARY

Cyclocryotherapy is one of a variety of cyclodestructive procedures now available to reduce intraocular pressure in patients who are not good candidates for filtration surgery. After retrobulbar anesthesia, 5 to 6 applications of 60-second duration at −80°C applied over 180° of the retrolimbal circumference completes the procedure. Transient uveitis invariably, and pain commonly, follow the procedure, but chronic uveitis, hypotony, and ciliochoroidal detachment occasionally occur.

BIBLIOGRAPHY

Bellows AR, Grant WM: Cyclocryotherapy in advanced inadequately controlled glaucoma. *Am J Ophthalmol* 1973;**75**:679–684.

Shields MB: Cyclodestructive surgery for glaucoma: past, present, and future. *Trans Am Ophthalmol Soc* 1985;**83**:285–303.

Commentary

Richard P. Mills, MD

I favor filtration enhancement over cyclodestruction whenever a patient has visual potential and the risk–benefit ratio to some form of filtration procedure is favorable. If postoperative hypotony occurs following cyclodestruction, it is irreversible and often leads to phthisis bulbi, whereas further surgery to limit outflow can in most cases reverse hypotony following filtration surgery.

As Dr Van Buskirk points out, cyclodestruction can be useful to reduce pain in blind glaucomatous eyes when enucleation is not desirable. With such patients, consideration should be given to injection of absolute alcohol in conjunction with the retrobulbar anesthetic. The severe pain often experienced for a few days following cyclocryotherapy is absent. The technique is to inject 2 to 3 ml 2% lidocaine, detach the syringe (leaving the retrobulbar needle in place for a few minutes while the anesthesia develops), and then inject 0.5 cc absolute ethanol into the same site.

After 180° of cyclodestruction, the intraocular pressure may not be sufficiently low and re-treatment is required. The risk of overtreatment can be reduced by overlapping 90° of the re-treatment with the previously treated area, thus treating only 90° of previously untreated ciliary body.

CHAPTER 18

Other Cyclodestructive Procedures

George Baerveldt, MD

For many years, cyclocryotherapy was the only cyclodestructive treatment available to ophthalmologists. The recent introduction of two new modalities capable of destroying the ciliary body and ciliary epithelium has prompted renewed interest in this area. Both therapeutic ultrasound and the thermal mode of the Nd:YAG laser appear to have results similar to those obtained with cyclocryotherapy. Compared with cyclocryotherapy, both modalities claim a significant reduction in postoperative pain.

18-1

THERAPEUTIC ULTRASOUND

High-intensity ultrasound is focused on the ciliary body through the therapeutic ultrasound transducer. The treatment is performed using the immersion technique with degassed water. The ultrasound transducer is aligned perpendicular to the eye, and the correct distance is provided by an A-scan. A coaxial light source is used for aiming and positioning the ultrasound transducer to an area 2.5 mm posterior to the limbus. Six 5-second applications of ultrasound are used. All patients receive local retrobulbar anesthesia, as with cyclocryotherapy.

Histologic studies of pig and rabbit eyes show late thinning of the sclera over the treated area, with destruction of the ciliary body and ciliary epithelium. These histologic studies indicate that the major mode of action is direct damage to the ciliary body and ciliary epithelium. Theoretically, the possibility exists of an increased uveoscleral outflow and drainage through the thinned sclera.

18-1-1 Results

Since 1981, when therapeutic ultrasound was introduced, the success of obtaining an intraocular pressure equal to or less than 25 mm Hg has been 72% for a single treatment and 6% for re-treatment. However, the success rate of achieving intraocular pressure of 21 mm Hg or less is lower. Following the procedure, some patients demonstrate substantial immediate increases in intraocular pressure, which must be controlled with osmotics. All patients demonstrate mild uveitis and iritis following treatment and respond to topical corticosteroids. A few patients develop severe, persistent uveitis that can ultimately lead to hypotony and decreased visual acuity. The thinning of the sclera is seen clinically, and approximately 20% of patients with congenital glaucomas develop pronounced scleral thinning with or without staphyloma as compared with less than 5% of the adult population. Visual acuity decreases, as after other cyclodestructive procedures, with 2 lines or more decrease found in approximately 30% of patients. If a patient moves during the procedure, lid or corneoscleral burns can occur.

18-2

Nd:YAG CYCLOPHOTOCOAGULATION

The ruby laser was used initially to perform successful cyclophotocoagulation. With the introduction of the Nd:YAG laser, transscleral cyclophotocoagulation has become popular.

Histologic studies have demonstrated that the ideal placement for the burns is 1.0 to 1.5 mm posterior to the limbus. Approximately 30% of the laser energy is absorbed by the conjunctiva and sclera, with the remaining energy concentrated on the ciliary body and ciliary epithelium. The lesions produced are more localized than the diffuse lesions caused by cyclocryotherapy. If the laser burn is applied less than 1.0 mm posterior to the limbus, more direct damage to the iris results, with bubble formation in the anterior chamber and increased uveitis. If the laser burns are applied 2.0 mm or more posterior to the limbus, the energy is concentrated on the pars plana.

At present, there are two methods of applying the laser energy. The first is through a slit lamp using the thermal or free-running mode of the Nd:YAG laser. Some lasers can retrofocus the Nd:YAG laser beam approximately 3.6 mm from the helium-neon focusing beam. This defocusing ability appears to concentrate the laser energy more efficiently on the ciliary processes. The other method is to use a fiberoptic system with a handpiece to place the probe directly on the conjunctiva over the ciliary body and treat transsclerally.

At present, no standard technique is widely used. The multiple studies that have been published use different parameters. Most studies have used 30 to 40 burns placed 1.0 to 3.0 mm posterior to the limbus for 360°. The energy levels have varied from 4 to 8 J. Each burn raises a small white conjunctival lesion. The higher the energy level, the whiter the lesion becomes. The method I employ is to pretreat the patient with 1 drop of apraclonidine 1% followed by retrobulbar anesthesia. A Shields lens is placed on the eye. The lens has 1-mm markings on the flange to facilitate exact placement of burns. When the flange is pushed against the conjunctiva, the conjunctiva can be blanched and less conjunctival reaction is observed. The Lasag Microruptor II is set at approximately 4.5 J and the retrofocus is set at 9, which is the maximum retrofocusing ability of the machine. The treatment area is 1.0 to 1.5 mm posterior to the limbus, and approximately 30 to 36 burns are placed 360°.

18-2-1 Results

The success rates of this procedure appear to be similar to those achieved with cyclocryotherapy. Neovascular glaucomas demonstrate a lower success rate, about 50% to 60%, with a higher incidence of hypotony and phthisis. Aphakic glaucomas with open angles, on the other hand, have a higher success rate and appear to have less overall phthisis. Success rates include multiple treatments and, in general, two treatments are required to achieve adequate intraocular pressure control, although as many as five treatments have been described. If after three treatment sessions the intraocular pressure is not controlled, other treatment modalities should be considered.

Intraocular pressure usually decreases 1 and 2 hours following the treatment. This is in marked contrast to the substantial increases in intraocular pressure that can occur for the first 48 hours after cyclocryotherapy and therapeutic ultrasound. This decrease of intraocular pressure usually is maintained for 1 week and then gradually decreases even more over time. If the treatment is unsuccessful, intraocular pressure usually starts rising at this time and will drift back toward the pretreatment level.

Immediately following the procedure, patients develop flare and cells in the anterior chamber. The amount of inflammation is usually less than with cyclocryotherapy. The majority of patients have minimal or no pain following this procedure. Certain patients do have considerable pain, which can last up to 1 week. Overall, the pain appears to be significantly less than that associated with cyclocryotherapy. The incidence of hyphemas, phthisis, and vitreous hemorrhages appears to be similar to that with cyclocryotherapy. There appears to be a definite decrease in the phthisis rate and in cataract formation compared with cyclocryotherapy. Long-term followup is not yet available on these patients.

Longer followup after this procedure is necessary. The advantages of decreased pain following this procedure, as compared with cyclocryotherapy, and the decreased inflammation have made this laser procedure attractive.

18-3

SUMMARY

Therapeutic ultrasound and the thermal mode of the Nd:YAG laser have acceptable success rates as compared with cyclocryotherapy. Both of these new modalities need long-term followup so that any late complications can be assessed. Both techniques require expensive and sophisticated machines. The significant reduction in pain following these treatments is appealing. If the phthisis rates remain low, these new treatment modalities may be used instead of cyclocryotherapy. At present, transscleral Nd:YAG cyclophotocoagulation is more appealing because of the immediate postoperative decrease in intraocular pressure, in contrast to the rise in pressure after cyclocryotherapy or therapeutic ultrasound, and the relatively mild inflammatory response. The minimal effect the Nd:YAG laser has on the integrity of the sclera is another factor, in contrast to the scleral thinning seen with therapeutic ultrasound.

BIBLIOGRAPHY

Devenyi RG, Trope GE, Hunter WH, et al: Neodymium:YAG transscleral cyclocoagulation in human eyes. *Ophthalmology* 1987;94:1519–1522.

Silverman RH, Vogelsang B, Rondeau MJ, et al: Therapeutic ultrasound for the treatment of glaucoma. *Am J Ophthalmol* 1991;111:327–337.

Commentary

Richard P. Mills, MD

Though the opportunity seldom arises because the conditions are fortunately rare, patients with congenital or traumatic aniridia have ciliary processes that are directly visible through the goniolens and are accessible to cyclophotocoagulation with the argon laser. During vitrectomy, the endophotocoagulator can treat ciliary processes pushed into direct view with scleral depression. The laser can be set on continuous exposure, and the beam used to "paint" each process to turn it gray and shrink it. Treatment must be heavy, but without producing tissue explosions, and 270° to 360° should be treated because some of the pars plicata in any region is inaccessible to the laser. Indications are the same as for other cyclodestructive procedures.

When the Lasag Nd:YAG thermal mode is used for cyclodestruction, the patient's eye is usually fixed in the primary position. The laser energy is thus directed tangentially, rather than perpendicularly through the sclera. Energy aimed 1.0 to 1.5 mm from the external limbus creates lesions in the ciliary body more posteriorly in the pars plicata, and the energy cone is well peripheral to the lens equator. On the other hand, energy delivered with the contact Nd:YAG system passes perpendicular to the sclera, so distances of treatment from the limbus are not comparable to noncontact systems, and the energy cone is angled differently.

Treatment parameters are still being established for both types of transscleral Nd:YAG cyclophotocoagulation, and long-term results are still being collected. Whether the detrimental effects on visual acuity observed after cyclocryotherapy will also be noted after Nd:YAG cyclodestruction is not known, but will have a strong bearing on the ultimate indications and cost–benefit ratios for the procedure.

Commentary

Richard A. Lewis, MD

The introduction of the fiberoptic probe for delivery of Nd:YAG laser transscleral cyclophotocoagulation has afforded greater opportunity for surgeons to perform cyclo-destructive procedures. Several of these fiberoptic devices have been FDA-approved for transscleral cyclophotocoagulation. After a retrobulbar injection, 32 burns are placed 1 to 2 mm posterior to the limbus for 360° without treating the horizontal areas (3- and 9-o'clock positions). The energy parameters are 7 W for 0.7 second.

The advantage of Nd:YAG cyclode-structive procedures over cyclocryotherapy is that the amount of postoperative pain and swelling is less. The fiberoptic system has some advantages over the slit lamp in that it can be applied to patients during surgery, under general anesthesia—a distinct advantage in young patients and others in whom retrobulbar anesthesia is not possible.

Long-term studies are under way to provide further understanding of this procedure and the specific indications for its use in the treatment of glaucoma.

Commentary

Robert N. Weinreb, MD

The indications for the cyclodestructive procedures discussed in this chapter are similar to those for cyclocryotherapy. I believe these procedures should be reserved for patients whose visual potential is less than 20/200 and those for whom filtration surgery has a poor prognosis. Indications include patients with neovascular glaucoma and iris neovascularization, those who have undergone multiple surgical procedures resulting in considerable scarring of the conjunctiva, patients with limited visual potential, patients with cicatrizing diseases of the conjunctiva or cornea, and patients who are surgical risks because of systemic disease. As these techniques become more widely used, treatment parameters should be refined and indications/contraindications more clearly elucidated.

Name _____

Address _____

City and State _____ Zip _____

Telephone (_____) _____ *Academy Member ID# _____
           area code

Your ID Number is located following your name on any Academy mailing label, in your Membership Directory, and on your Monthly Statement of Account.

CATEGORY 1 CME CREDIT FORM

Ophthalmology Monographs 4

Glaucoma Surgical Techniques

You may claim 1 hour of Category 1 Continuing Education Credit, up to a 25-hour maximum for each hour you spend studying this Ophthalmology Monograph. If you wish to claim continuing education credit for your study of this monograph, you must complete and return the self-study examination answer sheet on the back of this page, along with the following signed statement, to the Academy offices:

American Academy of Ophthalmology
P.O. Box 7424
San Francisco, CA 94120-7424
ATTN: Education Department

I hereby certify that I have spent _____ (up to 25) hours of study on the Ophthalmology Monograph *Glaucoma Surgical Techniques* and that I have completed the self-study examination. (The Academy *upon request* will send you a transcript of the credits listed on this form. You can check the box below if you wish credit verification now.)

☐ Please send credit verification now.

Signature _____   _____
                                                 Date

MONOGRAPH COMPLETION FORM

Ophthalmology Monographs 4

Answer Sheet for *Glaucoma Surgical Techniques*

Question	Answer					Question	Answer				
1	a	b	c	d	e	28	a	b	c	d	e
2	a	b	c	d	e	29	a	b	c	d	e
3	T	F				30	a	b	c	d	e
4	a	h	c	d	e	31	a	b	c	d	e
5	a	b	c	d	e	32	T	F			
6	a	b	c	d	e	33	a	b	c	d	e
7	a	b	c	d	e	34	a	b	c	d	e
8	a	b	c	d	e	35	a	b	c	d	e
9	a	b	c	d	e	36	a	b	c	d	e
10	a	b	c	d	e	37	a	b	c	d	e
11	a	b	c	d	e	38	a	b	c	d	e
12	a	b	c	d	e	39	a	b	c	d	e
13	T	F				40	a	b	c	d	e
14	T	F				41	a	b	c	d	e
15	a	b	c	d	e	42	a	b	c	d	e
16	a	b	c	d	e	43	a	b	c	d	e
17	a	b	c	d	e	44	a	b	c	d	e
18	a	b	c	d	e	45	a	b	c	d	e
19	a	b	c	d	e	46	a	b	c	d	e
20	a	b	c	d	e	47	a	b	c	d	e
21	a	b	c	d	e	48	a	b	c	d	e
22	a	b	c	d	e	49	a	b	c	d	e
23	a	b	c	d	e	50	a	b	c	d	e
24	a	b	c	d	e	51	a	b	c	d	e
25	a	b	c	d	e	52	T	F			
26	a	b	c	d	e	53	T	F			
27	a	b	c	d	e	54	a	b	c	d	e
						55	a	b	c	d	e

SELF-STUDY EXAMINATION

The self-study examination for *Glaucoma Surgical Techniques* consists of 55 multiple-choice and true-false questions and is intended for use *following* completion of the monograph. Questions are constructed so that there is one "best" answer. For each question, record your initial impression on the answer sheet by circling the appropriate letter. It is recognized that a disagreement about the optimal answer may occur despite the attempt to avoid ambiguous selections. A discussion of the most appropriate answer to each question follows the examination. Answers should not be consulted until the entire examination has been completed.

Chapter 1

1. The most common cause of filtration failure is

  a. vitreous incarcerated in the filter

  b. lens blocking the filter

  c. iris incarcerated in the filter

  d. episcleral fibrous proliferation

  e. healing of the sclera

2. Which of the following phases does *not* occur during wound healing?

  a. inflammation

  b. wound remodeling

  c. absence of scar tissue

  d. proliferation of fibroblasts

  e. wound contraction

3. Inflammation enhances   **T**   **F**
wound healing.

4. Which of the following is *not* a desirable effect when using cycloplegic agents following filtering surgery?

  a. Inflammation is increased.

  b. The pupil is dilated.

  c. The anterior chamber of an aphakic eye is deepened.

  d. There may be less leakage of plasma proteins into the eye.

  e. none of the above

Chapter 2

5. The ideal placement for a trabeculectomy is

a. superonasally in a phakic eye

b. at the 12-o'clock position

c. in one of the inferior quadrants

d. usually in one of the inferior quadrants in a pseudophakic eye

e. none of the above

6. During the course of dissecting a trabeculectomy flap, the surgeon should expect

a. the blue limbus boundary to be encountered posterior to its location at the scleral surface

b. Schlemm's canal to be posterior to the scleral spur

c. fewer Axenfeld's loops nasally than temporally

d. the sclera to be homogeneous in texture even anterior to the scleral spur

e. all of the above

7. In a narrow-angle eye, the surgeon should

a. not dissect farther into clear cornea before entering the anterior chamber than in an eye with a deeper anterior chamber

b. use a fornix-based flap

c. be particularly cautious about doing a basal iridectomy

d. avoid doing a peripheral iridectomy

e. none of the above

8. Anatomic differences between adults' and children's eyes include

a. less obvious or absent pannus in children

b. more easily torn (more delicate) tissues in children

c. thinner sclera in children

d. relatively thicker Tenon's capsule in children

e. all of the above

Chapter 3

9. Filtration surgery is indicated for most glaucoma patients who

a. have intraocular pressure above 23 mm Hg on maximum tolerable medical therapy

b. do not like eyedrops and have had failed laser surgery

c. are on maximum tolerable medical therapy, have had maximal laser benefit, and whose visual function is failing or is likely to fail

d. have intraocular pressure above 23 mm Hg on maximum tolerable medical therapy and have had laser surgery

e. have had failed medical and laser surgical therapy and have documented progressive deterioration

10. A contraindication to filtration surgery is

   a. a blind painful eye

   b. a blind painless eye

   c. an intraocular neoplasm

   d. poor patient hygiene

   e. all of the above

11. Interval changes in the optic disc are best appreciated

   a. stereoscopically, using the magnification of the slit lamp and an appropriate diagnostic lens

   b. using the binocular indirect ophthalmoscope

   c. using the monocular indirect ophthalmoscope

   d. using the direct ophthalmoscope

   e. using automated perimetry

12. Frequent reasons for considering a topical medication "not tolerable" include all of the following *except*

   a. severe systemic side effects

   b. inability to comply with prescribed regimen

   c. variable myopia

   d. eyes sting after instillation of drops

   e. allergic conjunctivitis

Chapter 4

13. With limbus-based trabeculectomy, it is best for the conjunctival incision to overlie the posterior edge of the scleral flap.   **T**   **F**

14. The peripheral iridectomy with trabeculectomy should be as small as possible.   **T**   **F**

Chapter 5

15. The most common cause of failure of filtration surgery occurs

   a. at the inner ostium of the sclerostomy site

   b. at the outer ostium of the sclerostomy site

   c. from an incomplete iridectomy

   d. at the conjunctiva–sclera interface

   e. from an encapsulated bleb

16. All of the following statements concerning the period after filtration surgery are true *except*

   a. Aqueous flow is necessary for the formation of a bleb.

   b. Vision is distorted from inflammation, hypotony, and a shift in the lens–iris diaphragm.

   c. The objective is to maintain a permanent fistula through sclera into the subconjunctival space.

   d. Cycloplegics are rarely necessary.

   e. Severe ocular pain is unusual.

17. An elevated bleb with high intraocular pressure is indicative of a(n)

   a. successful outcome

   b. choroidal effusion

   c. encapsulated bleb

   d. wound leak

   e. occluded fistula

18. A flat bleb with low intraocular pressure requires treatment with a(n)

   a. Nd:YAG laser directed at the iris

   b. Nd:YAG laser directed at the vitreous

   c. Nd:YAG laser directed at the anterior hyaloid

   d. ocular massage

   e. pressure patch

Chapter 6

19. Which of the following is(are) an advantage of a fornix-based conjunctival flap over a limbus-based flap?

   a. Exposure is better.

   b. The procedure is technically easier.

   c. After peritomy, conjunctiva is not manipulated until the end of the procedure, when it is reattached.

   d. all of the above

   e. none of the above

20. Which of the following statements concerning a fornix-based conjunctival flap is *not* true?

   a. It is more difficult to obtain a fluid-tight closure.

   b. The success rate is comparable to that with a limbus-based conjunctival flap.

   c. It can be used with a full-thickness procedure.

   d. Caution is necessary with adjunctive 5-fluorouracil use.

   e. all of the above

Chapter 7

21. The Watson trabeculectomy differs from the standard Cairns trabeculectomy in that it

   a. excises a scleral block, including the scleral spur

   b. does not utilize an iridectomy

   c. is a full-thickness procedure

   d. uses a fornix-based conjunctival flap

   e. functions as a cyclodialysis

22. Compared to the standard Cairns trabeculectomy, the Watson trabeculectomy has a higher incidence of

   a. vitreous loss

   b. postoperative hyphema

   c. flat filtration blebs

   d. hypotony

   e. cataract

Chapter 8

23. Full-thickness surgery is advantageous in all of the following conditions *except*

  a. limbal scarring

  b. secondary glaucoma with a high risk of failure

  c. low-tension glaucoma

  d. previous failed trabeculectomy

  e. thin or scarred sclera

24. In the late postoperative period, full-thickness surgery is often complicated by a(n)

  a. thin bleb

  b. flat anterior chamber

  c. choroidal effusion

  d. elevated intraocular pressure

  e. choroidal hemorrhage

25. All of the following statements concerning full-thickness surgery are true *except*

  a. Conjunctival closure occurs in two layers.

  b. A fornix-based conjunctival flap is preferred.

  c. A paracentesis tract allows access to the anterior chamber to deepen the chamber and to confirm patency of the sclerostomy.

  d. A laser sclerostomy may be performed ab interno or ab externo.

  e. Buttonholes of the conjunctiva must be closed at the completion of the surgery.

26. Full-thickness surgery involves all of the following *except*

  a. limbal dissection

  b. a triangular scleral flap

  c. sclerostomy

  d. iridectomy

  e. conjunctival closure

Chapter 9

27. The best choice for optical correction in combined cataract extraction and trabeculectomy is

  a. aphakic eyeglasses

  b. a contact lens

  c. an iris-plane intraocular lens

  d. a posterior chamber intraocular lens

  e. an anterior chamber intraocular lens

28. The combined cataract extraction and trabeculectomy procedure, compared to two-stage surgery,

  a. is less expensive for the patient

  b. provides more rapid visual rehabilitation

  c. tends to avoid the postoperative spike in intraocular pressure common to cataract surgery

  d. usually produces a flatter bleb

  e. all of the above

Chapter 10

29. Which of the following is *not* an effect of 5-fluorouracil?

a. inhibition of episcleral fibrous proliferation

b. inhibition of the enzyme thymidylate synthase and DNA synthesis

c. interference with the effects of steroids

d. possible association with corneal surface irregularities because of toxicity to the corneal epithelium

e. none of the above

30. With which of the following conditions is 5-fluorouracil contraindicated?

a. a previous failed filter

b. an aphakic eye

c. an eye with a history of uveitis and secondary angle-closure glaucoma

d. an eye with abnormal lid function, together with corneal and conjunctival disease

e. all of the above

31. The most common complication associated with the postoperative use of 5-fluorouracil is

a. cataract

b. increased intraocular pressure

c. corneal changes, including superficial punctate keratitis and filaments

d. cystoid macular edema

e. all of the above

32. Corneal changes associated   T   F
with the use of 5-fluorouracil following filtering surgery are not dose-dependent.

Chapter 11

33. A functioning Molteno implant

a. shows active transport of aqueous across the capsular wall

b. has equal pressures in the eye and in the bleb (capsule)

c. has one-way aqueous flow in the tube

d. has an epithelial lining around the plates and tube

e. has little bleb elevation in most cases

34. Complications unique to shunt devices include all of the following *except*

a. erosion of the tube through conjunctiva

b. blockage of the tube by vitreous, capsule, or fibrin

c. profound hypotony in the early postoperative period

d. corneal decompensation from tube-touch

e. a "hypertensive phase" in the 3- to 12-week postoperative period

35. An alternative to implanting a drainage device in a patient with intractable glaucoma is

a. subsequent trabeculectomy

b. trabeculectomy with 5-fluorouracil

c. cyclocryotherapy

d. no further surgery

e. all of the above

Chapter 12

36. Which of the following statements concerning trabeculectomy on an aphakic patient is *not* true?

    a. The surgeon should expect a high risk of vitreous loss, most likely at the time of iridectomy.

    b. The surgeon should consider using a support ring in case vitrectomy is needed.

    c. The risk of choroidal hemorrhage is higher than with a phakic patient.

    d. A retrobulbar anesthetic is contraindicated.

    e. all of the above

37. Postoperative hyphema after trabeculectomy

    a. is relatively common and usually trivial

    b. is best avoided by careful hemostasis during surgery

    c. may be related to systemic drugs such as aspirin used preoperatively

    d. may occur late due to the proliferation of capillaries around the filtering fistula boundary

    e. all of the above

38. The routine postoperative management of trabeculectomy should include

    a. cycloplegia to minimize the risk of ciliary spasm and a shallow or flat anterior chamber

    b. frequent visits during the first several weeks to titrate topical anti-inflammatory agents

    c. a fundus examination, especially if the anterior chamber is shallow

    d. frequent intraocular pressure measurements

    e. all of the above

39. During the postoperative period after trabeculectomy,

    a. severe pain is common during the first few hours or days

    b. inflammation in the conjunctiva diminishes continually

    c. intraocular pressure is always lower than preoperatively

    d. the resumption of carbonic anhydrase inhibitors is not desirable

    e. none of the above

Chapter 13

40. Which of the following is *not* a clinically identifiable manifestation of a failing bleb?

a. encapsulated bleb

b. tight scleral flap

c. scleral fibrosis

d. internal occluding membrane

e. conjunctival microcysts

41. Which of the following clinical manifestations is most amenable to laser therapy of the failing bleb?

a. encapsulated bleb

b. tight scleral flap

c. scleral fibrosis

d. internal occluding membrane

e. conjunctival microcysts

Chapter 14

42. Argon laser trabeculoplasty

a. works by opening holes through the trabecular meshwork

b. usually will control intraocular pressure sufficiently well to permit discontinuation of all topical or systemic drugs

c. works equally well regardless of patient age

d. is most useful in the elderly patient with chronic open-angle glaucoma as an alternative to carbonic anhydrase inhibitors or as a means of postponing more invasive therapy

e. none of the above

43. Argon laser trabeculoplasty works best in

a. chronic open-angle glaucoma

b. pseudoexfoliation syndrome and pigmentary glaucoma

c. glaucoma associated with uveitis

d. posttraumatic glaucoma with angle recession

e. none of the above

44. Complications of argon laser trabeculoplasty include

a. transient ocular hypertension almost always obvious within a few hours

b. corneal burns

c. transient changes in refractive error

d. transient uveitis

e. all of the above

45. Which of the following statements concerning postoperative care after argon laser trabeculoplasty is(are) *not* true?

a. Patients may be sent home immediately, and a followup exam arranged for 1 week later.

b. Intraocular pressure should be monitored for 1 to 3 hours.

c. Intraocular pressure should be checked at 24 hours.

d. Intraocular pressure may not stabilize for 4 to 6 weeks.

e. all of the above

Chapter 15

46. The Nd:YAG laser is advantageous compared to the argon laser in completing an iridotomy for all of the following reasons *except*

  a. fewer pulses

  b. less total energy

  c. effect on pupil shape

  d. iris bleeding

  e. patient access

47. The procedure to successfully complete a patent iridotomy requires all of the following *except*

  a. patient positioning

  b. pretreatment with a miotic and an anesthetic

  c. Goldmann contact lens

  d. high magnification of the slit lamp

  e. thin area of iris

Chapter 16

48. The type of laser surgery that is most often useful for treating neovascular glaucoma is

  a. laser trabeculoplasty

  b. goniophotocoagulation

  c. panretinal photocoagulation

  d. laser iridectomy

  e. pupilloplasty

49. Laser peripheral iridoplasty may be a useful adjunct in the treatment of

  a. nanophthalmos

  b. anatomic narrow angles requiring argon laser trabeculoplasty

  c. plateau iris syndrome

  d. an insufficient space between the iris and the cornea in laser peripheral iridectomy

  e. all of the above

50. Prior to photomydriasis for reduced vision in patients with miotic pupils, it is important to

  a. measure intraocular pressure

  b. perform gonioscopy

  c. perform visual fields

  d. establish improved vision after the use of mydriatrics

  e. photograph the optic nerve head

51. In the treatment of malignant aphakic or pseudophakic glaucoma, the Nd:YAG laser energy is focused on the

  a. trabecular meshwork

  b. peripheral iris

  c. anterior hyaloid membrane

  d. ciliary body

  e. pupillary border

Chapter 17

52. The cryoprobe should be   T   F
placed 5 mm posterior to
the corneoscleral limbus for
cyclocryotherapy.

53. Cyclocryotherapy has a   T   F
better prognosis for success
in an aphakic eye with an
open angle than with a
closed angle.

Chapter 18

54. The best location for placing burns
with Nd:YAG cyclophotocoagulation is

  a. at the corneal limbus

  b. 1.0 to 1.5 mm posterior to the
limbus

  c. over the pars plana

  d. over the ora serrata

  e. none of the above

55. Which of the following offers a potential advantage of Nd:YAG cyclophotocoagulation compared with cyclocryotherapy?

  a. less pain

  b. reduced rate of phthisis

  c. immediate postoperative decrease in
intraocular pressure

  d. reduced inflammation

  e. all of the above

ANSWERS AND DISCUSSION

These answers and explanations are to help you confirm that the reasoning you used in finding the most appropriate answer was correct. If you missed the question, the answer may help you to decide whether it was due to misinterpretation of the question or to poor wording. If, instead, you missed the question because of miscalculation or failure to recall relevant information, the answer and the explanation may help fix the principle in your memory.

Chapter 1

1. **Answer—d.** Glaucoma filtering operations fail for a variety of reasons, including all of the above. However, the most common finding with failed glaucoma filtering procedures is episcleral fibrous proliferation.

2. **Answer—c.** Inflammation, proliferation of fibroblasts (with wound contraction), and wound remodeling are the three overlapping phases associated with wound healing.

3. **Answer—T.** In general, inflammation is an essential part of wound healing.

4. **Answer—a.** Cycloplegic agents are thought to enhance the blood–aqueous barrier, with reduced anterior segment inflammation. Because the pupil is dilated, there are fewer posterior synechiae.

Chapter 2

5. **Answer—a.** Placement of the fistula superonasally in a phakic eye allows the maximum flexibility subsequently should cataract extraction become necessary. Usually, the surgeon can rotate the incision and avoid damage to the functioning filter. The fistula should not be placed at the 12-o'clock position because that compromises access to both upper quadrants. Inferior filtering surgery is less desirable because of difficulty with access (especially nasally) and because of probable increase in the rate of late infection.

6. **Answer—a.** The blue limbus boundary recedes deep to the surface, corresponding to the margin of the scleral sulcus. Schlemm's canal is anterior to (or partly overlying) the scleral spur. Axenfeld's loops are more numerous nasally than temporally. The texture of the sclera becomes looser as the dissection approaches the margin of the cornea.

7. **Answer—c.** Dissecting anteriorly into clear cornea in a narrow-angle eye will help avoid encountering ciliary processes during the iridectomy. The processes tend to be anteriorly displaced relative to their location in eyes with deep anterior chambers. The reasons to consider a fornix-based flap are speed and improved exposure. A basal iridectomy in a narrow-angle eye may include the tips of ciliary processes and provoke brisk bleeding. A peripheral iridectomy is necessary to prevent iris incarceration in the fistula and should be standard during filtering surgery in almost all patients. Exceptions include patients with anterior chamber lenses, the haptics of which prevent iris mobility in the area of the fistula.

8. **Answer—e.** The limbal tissues in children's eyes are more fragile and more easily torn or perforated than in adults' eyes. Wounds are more likely to leak, and scleral closure should be left tighter than in the average adult.

Chapter 3

9. **Answer—c.** Patients should have failed intraocular pressure control following laser surgery, if indicated, while on maximum tolerable medical therapy. Lack of control is determined on the basis of present or prior progression at the current pressure or a severely damaged optic disc not likely to tolerate the current pressure.

10. **Answer—e.** Some visual potential should be present to salvage with successful surgery. Risk of metastasis or endophthalmitis constitutes the reason for the other contraindications.

11. **Answer—a.** Disc changes are often subtle and require a binocular magnified view. Visual field changes do not always correlate with disc changes.

12. **Answer—d.** Minor annoyances associated with topical medication are often tolerable after the physician reassures the patient. More serious side effects or disabling visual disturbances frequently mandate discontinuation of a medication.

Chapter 4

13. **Answer—F.** If the conjunctival incision overlies the edge of the scleral flap, it is more likely to adhere and limit the bleb to an anterior position.

14. **Answer—F.** The iris should not be allowed to incarcerate in the fistula, so the iridectomy should be as broad as the deep scleral excision.

Chapter 5

15. Answer—d. This cause of failure can be avoided by postoperative intervention with ocular massage, anti-inflammatory medications (including 5-fluorouracil when indicated), and careful observation for postoperative complications. This statement is not meant to minimize the importance of careful surgical technique, including the scleral dissection, iridectomy, and meticulous conjunctival closure.

16. Answer—d. Cycloplegics are an integral part of postoperative management to relax the ciliary body, deepen the anterior chamber, and dilate the pupil.

17. Answer—c. A successful outcome is characterized by an elevated bleb with normal intraocular pressure. An elevated bleb with elevated intraocular pressure is described as encapsulated. This is most often a self-limited condition with a good prognosis. Patients who develop a choroidal effusion or a wound leak have low intraocular pressure. An occluded sclerostomy most often demonstrates a flat bleb and normal-to-elevated intraocular pressure.

18. Answer—e. A patient with a flat bleb and low intraocular pressure should be examined for a wound leak. The leak can be confirmed with a Seidel test using fluorescein and looking for aqueous flow. Initial treatment involves a pressure patch; a bandage contact lens, collagen shield, or Simmons shell is a good alternative. If unsuccessful, closure of the conjunctival wound with 10-0 nylon on a tapered needle is indicated.

Chapter 6

19. Answer—d. With less manipulation of conjunctiva, the surgeon is less likely to buttonhole the tissue.

20. Answer—c. Although the fornix-based flap can be employed with a full-thickness procedure, the propensity for wound leak and exposure makes it a relative contraindication.

Chapter 7

21. Answer—a. The deep scleral block is dissected from the posterior (overlying ciliary body) into clear cornea across the scleral spur. Despite early communication between the anterior chamber and the suprachoroidal space, cyclodialysis clefts do not persist postoperatively.

22. Answer—b. Hyphema is more common because of the more posterior dissection in the Watson trabeculectomy. Other complications occur at similar rates with either method.

Chapter 8

23. **Answer—a.** Full-thickness surgery is advantageous in producing greater lowering of intraocular pressure than does a trabeculectomy. It is particularly useful in patients with low-tension glaucoma and those with a high risk of failure. It is contraindicated in patients with conjunctival scarring at the limbus.

24. **Answer—a.** It is in the early postoperative period that many of the complications are encountered: flat anterior chamber, choroidal effusion, suprachoroidal hemorrhage, and hypotony. In the late postoperative period, the bleb tends to become thin and is more susceptible to infection.

25. **Answer—b.** A fornix-based flap is generally not preferred in full-thickness surgery because of the greater difficulty in achieving fluid-tight closure, without which the risk of a postoperative flat chamber, hypotony, and choroidal effusion is increased.

26. **Answer—b.** By definition, full-thickness surgery does not involve a scleral covering. The triangular flap is used in trabeculectomy, a partial-thickness procedure. The iridectomy is important because without it the sclerostomy site is often obstructed by adjacent iris.

Chapter 9

27. **Answer—d.** A posterior chamber intraocular lens provides the best protection of the corneal endothelium in the event of a shallow anterior chamber and a better optical result than either eyeglasses or a contact lens.

28. **Answer—e.** Single-stage surgery produces some efficiencies, although the quality of filtration is frequently less than that obtained with a two-stage operation.

Chapter 10

29. **Answer—c.** 5-Fluorouracil has several effects, including the inhibition of DNA and RNA synthesis with resulting inhibition of episcleral fibrous proliferation. As a consequence of its effects on DNA and RNA, it also appears to prevent corneal epithelial division.

30. **Answer—d.** Corneal and conjunctival disease, as well as lid exposure, increases the susceptibility of an eye to the toxic effects of 5-fluorouracil.

31. **Answer—c.** The earliest changes of 5-fluorouracil toxicity seem to be superficial punctate keratitis and filaments.

32. **Answer—F.** The presence of a corneal change should indicate the need for reducing the amount of 5-fluorouracil being delivered.

Chapter 11

33. Answer—b. Passive aqueous diffusion occurs across the capsular walls, which are collagenous tissue with no epithelial lining. Two-way flow keeps pressures equal in the eye and in the bleb.

34. Answer—e. Standard trabeculectomies may have a "hypertensive phase" associated with bleb encapsulation, which may spontaneously resolve.

35. Answer—e. Multiple options for such a patient exist and should be discussed when obtaining informed consent, including the option of no further intervention.

Chapter 12

36. Answer—d. The risk of vitreous loss is more likely in an aphakic patient because of the lack of a barrier between the vitreous cavity and the anterior chamber. Pseudophakic patients are not at great risk for vitreous loss during trabeculectomy unless the lens capsule or zonule was previously disrupted. A support ring is extremely helpful, especially for the solo surgeon if vitrectomy is required during filtering surgery in an aphakic patient. The sclera may collapse posteriorly during surgery, greatly complicating control of the wound. The risk of choroidal hemorrhage is higher in aphakic than phakic patients. There is no contraindication to the use of retrobulbar anesthetic in aphakia.

37. Answer—e. Mild postoperative hyphema is common after trabeculectomy and usually clears without special treatment. Massive bleeding can be disastrous, rarely requiring irrigation or reoperation. The preoperative history-taking should always include a query as to the use of vasoactive drugs, especially epinephrine or dipivefrin, and their elimination if possible for weeks before surgery. Anticoagulants are of obvious concern because they aggravate intraoperative or postoperative bleeding. Capillaries may proliferate along the margin of the scleral wound, visible gonioscopically, and bleed late after trabeculectomy. Microhyphema may be a cause of an otherwise-unexplained rise in intraocular pressure late in the postoperative period despite an apparently functional filter.

38. Answer—e. Cycloplegia, preferably with atropine, is extremely important to minimize ciliary spasm and shallowing of the anterior chamber. Any degree of shallowing of the anterior chamber should prompt a fundus examination with indirect ophthalmoscopy to exclude choroidal detachment or choroidal hemorrhage. Detachment of the ciliary body is often the best explanation for shallowing of the anterior chamber. Overfiltration through the fistula is usually associated with a huge bleb, often expanding around the circumference of the limbus. Compression of the trabeculectomy flap at the slit lamp will sometimes produce rapid deepening of the anterior chamber if overfiltration is responsible for the shallow chamber. Significant pain postoperatively should raise concern about a choroidal hemorrhage. If the fundus cannot be seen, ultrasound is indicated.

39. **Answer—d.** Pain after filtering surgery is a bad sign and often indicates choroidal hemorrhage. This complaint should stimulate a thorough examination, including funduscopy and ultrasound if necessary. Shallowing of the anterior chamber and hyphema may occur as a complication of choroidal hemorrhage. The inflammatory reaction in the conjunctiva is usually maximal about 3 to 4 weeks after filtering surgery, at which time intraocular pressure may rise. Continued or increased use of topical steroids is usually indicated. Intraocular pressure will often fall during the subsequent weeks unless a cystic, impermeable bleb forms or the patient is a steroid responder. Ocular massage and resumption of a beta blocker may be indicated. Resumption or use of carbonic anhydrase inhibitors is probably undesirable but may be necessary depending on intraocular pressure and the state of the optic nerve in the operated or other eye.

Chapter 13

40. **Answer—e.** Conjunctival microcysts are an indication of bleb function and should be searched for.

41. **Answer—d.** The Nd:YAG laser is directed gonioscopically to re-establish aqueous flow. The other causes of bleb failure are not easily approached with the laser.

Chapter 14

42. **Answer—d.** The mechanism by which argon laser trabeculoplasty effects a drop in intraocular pressure is not known. Most likely the application of laser energy to the meshwork produces a contraction (tightening) of trabecular beams. A longer-lasting effect may be due to repair of injured trabecular endothelium. Migration of corneal endothelium into injured areas of meshwork may explain the findings by scanning electron microscopy, suggesting fusion of trabecular beams at the site of the burns. Argon laser trabeculoplasty has a higher success rate in patients over 50 years of age. It seldom works well enough to permit discontinuation of all topical or systemic medications.

43. **Answer—b.** Argon laser trabeculoplasty has been recognized since its first application to clinical glaucoma to work relatively well in pseudoexfoliation and pigmentary glaucomas. The explanation for the relatively better success in these conditions is unknown. ALT has not worked well in posttraumatic glaucoma and is contraindicated in glaucoma associated with uveitis.

44. Answer—e. The primary complication of ALT is transient rise in intraocular pressure, almost always obvious by 1 to 2 hours after the procedure. Recent use of apraclonidine as pretreatment has virtually eliminated the problem of very high intraocular pressure. Alternatives to apraclonidine include additional miotic instillation, alcohol, and hyperosmotic agents. Transient rise in intraocular pressure may be associated with "snuff-out" of optic nerve function in patients with advanced optic nerve injury. Besides transient rise in intraocular pressure, corneal (both epithelial and endothelial) burns, transient change in refractive error, and iritis may occur. Later complications include characteristic focal peripheral anterior synechiae after burns that were too intense and too posterior.

45. Answer—a. Ideally, patients should be treated with ALT during the morning hours to permit 1 to 3 hours of follow-up in the clinic to monitor intraocular pressure. The risk of transient elevation of intraocular pressure is greatly minimized by the preoperative use of apraclonidine. Intraocular pressure may become elevated several hours after ALT, and rarely spikes after 12 to 24 hours. The hazard of a transient rise in intraocular pressure varies with the status of the optic nerve in the eye being treated. In end-stage disease, it is important to monitor intraocular pressure carefully. The final pressure after ALT may not become apparent until 4 to 6 weeks postoperatively. There is no correlation established between the immediate response of intraocular pressure following ALT and long-term results.

Chapter 15

46. Answer—d. The Nd:YAG is portable and requires less energy and fewer pulses. However, bleeding is more likely with the Nd:YAG laser than with the argon laser.

47. Answer—c. The procedure is facilitated with the aid of a special iridotomy lens, which is a high-power, planoconvex lens affixed to a contact lens. The use of such a lens prevents corneal burns, controls eye movement, and aids in lid retraction.

Chapter 16

48. Answer—c. Therapy of neovascular glaucoma should be directed at curtailing the stimulus for neovascularization by ablating the ischemic retina via panretinal photocoagulation, cryoablation, or endophotocoagulation during vitreous surgery. Goniophotocoagulation is used as a temporary measure in patients who are receiving or have recently received ablation to the ischemic retina.

49. Answer—e. Peripheral iridoplasty is a very useful procedure by which the configuration of the peripheral iris can be changed. This can be therapeutic in the treatment of nanophthalmos and plateau iris syndrome or adjunctive prior to argon laser trabeculoplasty in anatomic narrow angles or laser peripheral iridectomy in narrow or closed angles.

50. Answer—d. Photomydriasis can be used to enlarge miotic pupils in patients with developing cataracts. It is very important to establish a subjective improvement in vision using mydriatics prior to proceeding with laser photomydriasis.

51. Answer—c. In aphakic or pseudophakic malignant glaucoma, the anterior hyaloid membrane acts as a barrier to the forward flow of aqueous into the anterior segment. It is possible to release this block by disrupting the anterior hyaloid and anterior vitreous with the Nd:YAG laser, creating a passageway between the trapped aqueous and the anterior segment.

Chapter 17

52. Answer—F. The pars plicata of the ciliary body is located 0.5 to 2.5 mm posterior to the limbus. The cryoprobe should be centered 1.5 to 2.0 mm posterior to the limbus for maximal effect, while sparing the peripheral corneal endothelium.

53. Answer—T. A closed angle has so little outflow that the inflow must be titrated more delicately than is usually possible with cyclocryotherapy.

Chapter 18

54. Answer—b. The pars plicata of the ciliary body is centered 1.0 to 1.5 mm behind the limbus.

55. Answer—e. Reduced pain in the immediate postoperative period relates to the lower intraocular pressure and less inflammation observed following laser cyclodestruction. Whether the rate of phthisis will remain lower with longer followup is still not known.

INDEX

NOTE: A *t* following a page number indicates tabular material, and an *f* following a page number indicates an illustration. Drugs are listed under their generic names; when a drug trade name is listed, the reader is referred to the generic name.

A

Abraham laser iridotomy lens, 128, 131
Alpha adrenergic agents, in argon laser trabeculoplasty, 119
ALT. *See* Argon laser, for trabeculoplasty
Anesthesia
    for argon laser trabeculoplasty, 119
    for cyclocryotherapy, 143
    for laser iridotomy, 127
Angiogenesis inhibitors, wound healing affected by, 6
Anterior chamber, after filtration surgery
    late bleeding into, 92
    shallow or flat, 93
Anterior chamber lens, in combined glaucoma and cataract surgery, 61
Anterior segment. *See also* Limbus
    anatomic features of, 8–14
    after trabeculectomy, 38–39
Antibiotics, after trabeculectomy, 35–36
Antifibroproliferative agents (antiproliferative agents)
    after combined glaucoma and cataract surgery, 71
    wound healing and, 6
Anti-inflammatory drugs, for encapsulated bleb, 101
Antimetabolites, filtration surgery and, 72–76
    complications of, 74–75, 75–76
    indications for, 72–73, 76
    postoperative care and, 73–74, 75–76, 76
    preoperative considerations in use of, 72–73
    surgical technique and, 73
    wound closure and, 73, 76
Antiproliferative agents (antifibroproliferative agents)
    after combined glaucoma and cataract surgery, 71
    wound healing and, 6

Aphakic eyes
    drainage sites in, 12
    Molteno implant placement in, 81
    Nd:YAG laser photocoagulation in, 138–139, 140
Apraclonidine
    in argon laser trabeculoplasty, 119, 122, 125
    before laser iridotomy, 128, 132
Aqueous leak, after filtration surgery, 94
Aqueous misdirection, after filtration surgery, 95–96
Argon laser
    in epithelial downgrowth, 141
    for goniophotocoagulation, 137, 140
    for gonioplasty, 133–134, 140
    for iridotomy, 127–132
        complications of, 130
        indications for, 127
        vs Nd:YAG laser, 132
        postoperative care and, 130
        results of, 129
        surgical technique for, 127–129, 131
    miscellaneous uses of, 133–141
    for peripheral iridoplasty, 133–134, 140
    for photocoagulation in malignant glaucoma, 138
    for photomydriasis, 135, 140
    for pupilloplasty, 134
    for shrinking conjunctival blebs, 141
    for sphincterotomy, 135
    for tight scleral flap lysis, 110, 111*f*, 116, 136